Masterpieces in

HEALTH CARE LEADERSHIP

Cases and Analysis for Best Practice

Editors

VINCE PELOTE, MBA
PARTNER
DAVINCI CONSULTING

LYNNE ROUTE, RN, BSN, MEd
PARTNER
DAVINCI CONSULTING

Contributing Editor

MARY MALONE, JD
PRESIDENT
MALONE ADVISORY SERVICES

JONES AND BARTLETT PUBLISHERS
Sudbury, Massachusetts
BOSTON   TORONTO   LONDON   SINGAPORE

World Headquarters

Jones and Bartlett Publishers	Jones and Bartlett Publishers	Jones and Bartlett Publishers
40 Tall Pine Drive	Canada	International
Sudbury, MA 01776	6339 Ormindale Way	Barb House, Barb Mews
978-443-5000	Mississauga, Ontario	London W6 7PA
info@jbpub.com	L5V 1J2	UK
www.jbpub.com	CANADA	

Jones and Bartlett's books and products are available through most bookstores and online booksellers. To contact Jones and Bartlett Publishers directly, call 800-832-0034, fax 978-443-8000, or visit our website, www.jbpub.com.

Substantial discounts on bulk quantities of Jones and Bartlett's publications are available to corporations, professional associations, and other qualified organizations. For details and specific discount information, contact the special sales department at Jones and Bartlett via the above contact information or send an email to specialsales@jbpub.com.

Copyright © 2007 by Jones and Bartlett Publishers, Inc.

All rights reserved. No part of the material protected by this copyright may be reproduced or utilized in any form, electronic or mechanical, including photocopying, recording, or by any information storage and retrieval system, without written permission from the copyright owner.

Production Credits
Publisher: Michael Brown
Production Director: Amy Rose
Production Assistant: Amy Browning
Marketing Manager: Sophie Fleck
Associate Editor: Katey Birtcher
Manufacturing Buyer: Therese Connell
Composition: Northeast Compositors, Inc.
Cover Design: Timothy Dziewit
Cover Image: © Marc Dietrich/ShutterStock, Inc.
Printing and Binding: Malloy, Inc.
Cover Printing: Malloy, Inc.

Library of Congress Cataloging-in-Publication Data
Masterpieces in health care leadership : cases and analysis for best practice / [edited by] Vince Pelote and Lynne Route.
     p. ; cm.
  Includes bibliographical references.
  ISBN-13: 978-0-7637-3880-8
  ISBN-10: 0-7637-3880-8
  1. Health services administration. 2. Health services administration—Case studies. I. Pelote, Vincent P. II. Route, Lynne.
  [DNLM: 1. Health Services Administration. 2. Leadership. 3. Personnel Management—methods. 4. Staff Development—methods. W 84.1 M423 2007]
  RA971.M39 2007
  362.1068—dc22
                                        2007005822

6048

Printed in the United States of America
11 10 09 08 07   10 9 8 7 6 5 4 3 2 1

DEDICATION

To my mom and dad, who led me to my reward.
And to my girls, Brie, Gabe, and Sam, whom I hope to inspire
to follow their dreams.

—Lynne

To my mom, Rose, who has always believed in me.

—Vince

Table of Contents

Introduction

This is a book of power. When we say power we are referring to powerful actions that positively impact others and to the use of power to influence others at very deep levels. We have a lifelong passion to help others in terms of what they want to achieve and aspire to.

We did not want to write a book of solutions—the shelves are already filled with extremely well-written "how-to" works. We did not see ourselves as the experts who would provide well-defined solutions to problems. Our book, *Masterpieces in Health Care Leadership: Cases and Analysis for Best Practice,* does not include methods for reducing days in your billing process or provide guidance on how to redesign your new employee orientation. Rather, it is a collection of powerful and compelling stories of how leaders have engaged their staff members to improve the billing cycle or to develop a new employee orientation.

Our ultimate goal for this book of power was to explore these questions: How can we help others? How can we have an impact in healthcare? We surmised that the answers existed with those who were already successful. There are exemplary healthcare organizations and leaders who are achieving extraordinary results. Our mission was to showcase these organizations and their leaders and to share their stories.

By sharing these examples in their purest form, we hoped we could have a positive impact. We chose to share these successes through positive and powerful stories. We were comfortable knowing that others could learn what had been accomplished and what successful practices were emerging through the stories of successful leaders. Ultimately, we found that the entire mental model of storytelling is, in itself, a new and emerging way of leading. Although we wanted to write a book about power, we discovered that we were also writing a book about leadership.

In contrast to the current mental model, we discovered that the new leaders, the masterpiece leaders, spent most of their time focusing on behavioral competencies that rest within the domain of power. Instead of focusing on coming up with creative ideas, analyzing details, establishing productive teams, maintaining integrity, and remaining flexible (the time our masterpiece leaders spent on these behaviors was minimal), masterpiece leaders spent most of their time in less concrete domains. They spent most of their time leading others, impacting and influencing others, developing others, and working to make things better. These leaders also spent less than half of their time on customer service focus, change leadership, relationship building, information seeking, and inquiry. We have observed that the result of the time spent in those power domains had a positive effect on the climate of the workers, as evidenced by the comments and stories from staff and patient interviews.

This book explains these findings in detail and provides numerous examples of those actions in the form of stories spoken in the participants' own words. In addition, this book explains the process in which we uncovered those stories, how we identified those distinctive behaviors, and how resultant conclusions and implications may impact others.

And so in writing this book about power we also wrote a book about leadership.

Foreword

Health care continues to be among the most pressing challenges of the 21st century. Across the United States, we experience not only a crisis of care but also a crisis of organization. The very institutions whose job it is to organize services, to deliver care, and to ensure well-being for the people of our country are themselves in ill health. Costs continue to rise. The delivery of service depends on an overly complex balance of high technology, high touch, and extensive administration. Quality care is elusive to many who need it. As people in need have more access to information via the Internet and yet have less access to actual care, frustration with healthcare leadership rises.

Add to this the changing population demographics, respective changes in services needed and wanted, increasing numbers of diseases with epidemical potential, decreasing numbers of healthcare professionals in crucial areas, increasing interest in alternative health care and engagement in the healing process, and we have a situation ripe with potential—a healthcare system in need of great attention and leadership.

Given the challenges of the time, to produce a book on healthcare leadership is both a courageous and also a profoundly important task. The editors and authors of this book have taken a bold stand. In an age of disenfranchisement with health care, they have sought to discover and share the appreciative alternatives. By seeking out and studying healthcare institutions that are succeeding and by making their stories known, they offer hope for the future.

This book contains both visions of possibility and paths forward. It is a wealth of information in the form of stories about how to excel in health care today. Woven throughout the book is the message that no matter what else they do, leaders must be role models. At Clinton, "The hands-on leadership and role-modeling demonstrated by the unit leader and her attention to helping the staff members keep a good balance between their work lives and personal lives have a positive impact on the team members." At RWJUH-H, the message is to be a role model with humility, "Leaders are role models—approachable, humble, exemplars—and yet take responsibility for the ultimate results. At the same time, they exercise great humility and make great efforts to share the recognition and awards with team members." At Mountain States, "The leaders appear extraordinarily self-aware that what they do is as important as what they say. They set the example of the vision of the organization and role model the expected behaviors. They practice what they preach."

To be a masterpiece of leadership in health care today is not a simple task. As the story from Greenwich shows, success requires attention to a complex set of variables, including service standards, management structures, and celebrations. "The meaningful connection of the service standards (expectations) to employee evaluations and compensation at 60% is quite a statement. . . . The linkage of the performance goals (in service and everywhere else) to the money put into the retirement fund is a brilliant strategy. . . . It starts with the Wednesday meeting—led by the CEO and COO—which reviews all of the input from patients, families, visitors, and community members received during the past week. The expectation of remedial action and accountability for results by the next week's meeting is extraordinary. . . . Celebrations of all sorts—formal and informal—provide inspiration and appreciation to the staff. These contribute to the development of teamwork and trust that is essential to their ongoing success."

Perhaps the most significant message carried by the stories in this book is that when employees are truly valued and cared for, they in turn value and care for clients and patients. At the Cleveland Clinic, "Their philosophy of connecting to each employee's individual mission has had a powerful impact. The effect on the employees, as told in stories, has been as transformative for them, as it has been on the patients, families, and nurses who are their customers." The extraordinary story of the Cathedral Foundation says it most clearly: When leaders develop people, their clients and organizations benefit. "Human potential—whether that of the resident or the employee—is valued, developed, and encouraged throughout Cathedral. The leaders provide the support that employees need to be successful in their current jobs and are given the confidence to learn and grow in their personal and professional lives. . . . The care that leaders take in selecting the right employees is apparent in several stories. While it might seem expedient to take 'the next warm body,' the leaders are committed to making sure that they have the right person for the job. Their commitment to developing human potential even extends to those applicants that they don't hire by letting them know they will be successful somewhere else even if they aren't a good fit for this position."

As this book illustrates, masterpieces in health care abound. This book can help you and your organization be one. Just as medications work when they are taken, the wisdom of this book will help cure the ills of your organizations only if you apply it in real and tangible ways. I suggest you take a dose of this book, read it, and find the stories that most resonate with your current situation. Borrow and adapt the best ideas and make them your own. When you succeed, tell your story—keep the best ideas flowing. We cannot afford to be greedy with best practices in health care. This book sets us on a course of generosity, of sharing what works. It is an act of leadership worthy of emulation.

Diana Whitney
Taos, New Mexico

Preface

BIRTH OF A MASTERPIECE

Through years of research in the behavioral sciences and careers in health care, we learned fascinating things about leaders and healthcare leadership. We continually asked, "How can we use this knowledge and experience to help others in the healthcare field?"

A presentation by Don Berwick helped to frame our thinking. Berwick, president, CEO, and cofounder of the Institute for Healthcare Improvement in Boston, referred to the importance of positive questions. He said, "One of the things that is missing in healthcare is that we're not asking the right questions." He also said that we are not learning from people that are already doing it well. Those statements provided the direction for this book. We needed to ask really good questions of those who were successful. It struck a chord with us, and we started asking ourselves, "To whom do we need to ask questions? What do we need to ask them?"

We explored the concept of appreciative inquiry and began to use this approach with our clients. We asked appreciative questions and incorporated the stories we gathered as part of our presentations and workshops. Asking those positive questions and having participants share their own positive stories made our workshops come alive.

As we delved into this new approach we made other discoveries. We found that we were intrigued by Leonardo da Vinci's approach of getting deep behind the science of the human body in order to create artistic masterpieces. We thought his combination of art and science was brilliant! Da Vinci dissected the layers of the human form and studied anatomy in depth in order to understand its underpinnings. In doing so, he made the human form come alive with motion in a manner that amazed his contemporaries and continues to capture others today.

We drew the parallel that understanding human behavior at a deep level would lead to creating masterpieces in leadership and make those come alive. As our discussion evolved, we became increasingly excited and inspired. We felt that healthcare leaders needed to venture outside of the constructs of their traditional training and profession to other communities of practice so that they might better understand the underpinnings of organizational dynamics. We felt that these explorations were key in creating successes in healthcare leadership.

When visiting the Brigham & Women's Hospital in Boston, we were struck by the greatness of the *Healers of Our Age* photographic exhibit. Here were larger-than-life portraits of individuals such as Albert Einstein and Carl Jung. We wanted to learn more about the person who had taken these photographs. Yousuf Karsh was one of the most renowned portrait photographers of the 20th century. To our delight, Yousuf & Estrellita Karsh were longtime supporters of Brigham & Women's Hospital. Estrellita Karsh was someone very special—someone who was not only interested in sharing the work of her late husband but who also genuinely wanted to help us with our work. Through her constant encouragement, generosity, and patience, we have come to understand and appreciate Yousuf Karsh's unique and enduring way of building relationships with his photographic subjects. We learned much about connecting with others and establishing relationships. Here was another example of a great master who combined art and science.

Several of Karsh's statements had a profound impact on us and guided us in further defining our approach. The first was about creating a truthful portrait: "Sometimes we meet for ten minutes, sometimes for two hours, and in that time it is my task to produce of my sitter an image that is true, not merely fleeting but that man's inner life, his strength and weakness, a picture that will show with equal force his past, present, and even something of his future" (Karsh, 1957). Karsh also said about power: "The endless fascination of these people for me lies in what I call their inward power. It is part of the elusive secret that hides in everyone, and it has been my life's work to try to capture it on film. The mask we present to others and, too often to ourselves may lift for only a second—to reveal that power in an unconscious gesture, a raised brow, a surprised response, a moment of repose. This is the moment to record" (Karsh, 2003).

As we were exploring da Vinci and Karsh's approaches, an earlier event resurfaced as an epiphany. While sitting on a tour bus headed for the Uffizi gallery in Florence, the tour guide posed the following question: "Does anybody know the difference between a great work of art and a masterpiece?" The answer was: "The difference is passion. A great work of art is commissioned. A masterpiece is created out of passion."

Early on in this project we discovered that all the successful leaders we interviewed shared one common thread: passion. We had come full circle. Here we were back to that word passion. If we connected the passion of the leaders with the behavioral sciences at work behind their leadership, we would uncover that translation we were looking for. If we presented it through a positive lens, the masterpiece would be there for others to see and benefit from. Albert Einstein said it best in his words to Karsh: "In art, and in the higher ranges of science, there is a feeling of harmony, which underlines all endeavor. There is no true greatness in the art of science without that sense of harmony. He who lacks it can never be more than a great technician in either field" (Karsh, 1971).

That was the birth of our masterpiece project.

Acknowledgments

Lynn Dalbec, whose transcription provided an accurate account of our interviews and who worked tirelessly through the nights.

Matthew Zirakian for capturing our Masterpiece Summit with photographs and audio recoding.

Gabriella LaMonica and Julianne Mazzawi, our student interns, for their behind-the-scenes work with data input, report generating, and support at our Masterpiece Summit.

Diana Whitney for writing our foreword and coaching us through our manuscript preparation.

Patty Segerson for reading our work and providing feedback.

Ian Copland for his analysis of climate and BEI data and for graphic presentation of our data.

Shirley Tierney for her work in recreating the leadership competency and style analysis and for graphic presentation of our data.

Our organizational contacts:

Christine Beechner, Greenwich Hospital
Sharon Brown, The Cathedral Foundation
Charlene Elie, Clinton Hospital
Dianne Grillo, Robert Wood Johnson University Hamilton
Randy Hutchison, Geisinger Health System
Joel Katz, MD, Brigham & Women's Hospital
Sonia Rhodes, Sharp HealthCare
Tom Tull, Mountain States Health Alliance
Susan West, Fairview Hospital

Susan Wood for her participation, guidance, and insight in planning the Masterpiece Summit.

Paulette Seymour-Route for her research with Cathedral Foundation.

Allan Brownsword for his research with Geisinger Health System.

Judy Theisen for her timely chapter edits.

Sarah Pelote for her research and data entry.

Lyle Spencer for sharing his profound knowledge and mentoring around leadership competencies.

Ron Crandall for his valued friendship, continuous feedback, and reading our work.

Estrellita Karsh for her endless inspiration and guided tours of Yousuf Karsh's portraits.

All those individuals who shared their stories with us: leaders, staff, and patients.

CHAPTER 1

Background

MASTERPIECES IN HEALTHCARE LEADERSHIP

We refer to this book as a masterpiece project—not because we have created a masterpiece per se, but because we present a collection of masterpieces created by others. We posit that the differentiating factor in creating a masterpiece is passion. The organizations featured in this book (we call them the Masterpiece organizations) have attained measurable success in leading their organizations. Their success is driven by a similar passion.

EXEMPLARS

When we initially started talking about masterpieces, we considered "case studies" as a method for studying success. Many successful organizations had already been identified. Publications describing successful leadership had been published. We challenged ourselves to answer the following questions: What was the correlation between the two? How could we present that correlation in a new way that would be easy for others to understand? We quickly realized that a pure case study would be investigative but not interpretive. Cases would certainly describe the road to success but they would not illustrate the correlation between leadership and success at a practical level. We needed to present *examples* of the precise behaviors that translated into success. At this point we knew our chapters needed to be exemplars rather than case studies. In a dictionary, we stumbled on a definition of exemplar that really excited us: "Worthy of imitation." If we uncovered a collection of exemplars that were worthy of imitation, then perhaps others would be able to imitate those.

We decided the exemplars should be presented in the participants' own words. We did not want to add expertise. We did not want to "doctor-up" the examples to make the sentences sound better; we wanted to present them so that others would hear it like it was spoken. We wanted the true picture that Karsh sought (as described in the preface to this book). If people were to understand the underpinnings of success, then they needed to understand the true person and intent of their actions.

We asked ourselves further, "How can we make these examples usable and practical without interpretation and explanation?" That was when we realized that we needed to create a book of stories. If we looked at the hopes and the dreams of successful leaders and examined the thought–action sequencing behind their behaviors we would uncover explicit examples worthy of imitation. These examples, or stories, would be a wonderful blend of art and science and their impact would potentially be great.

Our journey became more solidified in terms of the stories after we interviewed folks in the pilot organization. When we heard the stories from the voices of the leaders and also the stories from the staff, the patients, and the stakeholders, we knew that we needed to share those examples. Their stories said it all. When we first heard them, we could not wait to share them with each other! When we did share, the impact was incredible. We felt their passion and it was contagious for them and us.

The passion came across on three levels: how they led their staff and cared for patients, how they were excited about sharing, and the way they shared. They did not simply report what they did; instead, they shared their feelings. They shared things that even they were not aware of, and the masterpiece became brilliant. The way they described it through their stories truly set them apart. The storytelling allowed their passion and true intent to be framed.

As we moved forward, this fervor continued to amaze us. These successful behaviors were modeled throughout each organization. The exemplars had no demographic boundaries. Whether we interviewed a midlevel manager or senior leader, a large conglomerate, or small department, the stories, the behaviors, and the passion were pervasive.

IDENTIFYING MASTERPIECE ORGANIZATIONS

We decided our masterpiece book would consist of a collection of stories from organizations that had already demonstrated success in the areas of patient satisfaction, employee engagement, and innovation in leadership. As you read these chapters, these topics will become apparent. Fortunately, as researchers, archeologists, and anthropologists, we were able to enlist nine exemplar organizations who were willing to share their thoughts, values, hopes, and dreams with us. Within our masterpiece organizations, we reveal those qualities through different perspectives and cross-sections of healthcare: some big and some small, some with a lot of capital and resources, and some with minimal resources. These organizations and the units and departments we interviewed, represent a diverse geography and unique vertical cross-sections of healthcare.

INVITING CONTRIBUTORS

In order to stay within our goal approach of presenting leadership behaviors that transcended all boundaries and in an effort to reach a broad audience, we did not want to present these remarkable stories strictly from our own perspective. We explored ways to interpret and present our research with the mindset: explore widely in order to reach many. We decided that we would enlist qualified individuals from different walks of life to assist in conducting our research and help us extract those pieces of research that they determined relevant.

When we were looking at selecting contributors, we wanted those who had zeal for their work. We wanted professionals from a variety of backgrounds—not just healthcare—who would use different lenses to focus on those stories that revealed success. We evaluated each candidate to see whether he or she was excited about going on this masterpiece journey. As a result, we enlisted contributors with backgrounds in healthcare, organizational development, academia, change leadership, appreciative inquiry, management consulting, and manufacturing.

DETERMINING PARTICIPANTS AND INTERVIEW SUBJECTS

When we realized that the same successful behaviors were apparent at all levels of the organizations, we decided that this book might appeal to all levels of leaders including CEOs and shift supervisors. Although job titles and roles differed, all could benefit from these exemplars.

We immediately started to develop an eclectic picture of where the stories would be collected from. In order to reach a diverse audience, we needed to direct our focus in different directions in each organization.

As we developed questions for the interviews, we tested all of these concepts with a pilot organization. We asked ourselves these questions: What did we want to know? Would the questions we created uncover what we hoped they would? Were we interviewing the right mix of people? We needed a vertical slice of the organization that could get at one focus area within the organization. In our pilot, it was the emergency department. We needed to find out whether the vertical slice was going to give us helpful information. How do we get a good representative sample? We knew we would look at the senior leadership and the emergency department leadership and patients from that area. We knew we needed to interview staff—but who within the staff? We knew we needed nurses; however, should we include other staff who interact within the department, such as, physicians, radiology technicians, and lab technicians? We knew also that there were stakeholders to interview. We asked the organization to help us identify them—in this case the referring physicians and the EMTs.

We sought to hear candidly what was going on from each of their perspectives. We wanted to hear responses to these questions: What did it feel like to work there if you're an EMT? What did it feel like to be a new employee? What did it feel like to be a patient? We wanted to know in its purest form: What were the hopes and dreams of the leaders and employees and what was the thought–action sequencing behind the behaviors? Thus, the pilot organization helped us uncover the right mix of participants that gave us a representative sample to uncover the essence of the organization.

We used the pilot organization to guide us through the remainder of the masterpiece project: using the assessment and climate tools, conducting the interviews, writing the exemplar chapters, and coaching our contributors through that process.

DESIGNING THE RESEARCH METHODS

We selected a variety of research methods to collect our data. Our approach would yield both qualitative and quantitative data—some self-reported and some empirical. We selected the healthcare climate survey, leadership self-assessment, social motive self-assessment, appreciative inquiry interviews, and behavioral event interviews. The leadership assessment consisted of two parts: leadership competency behaviors and leadership style.

We made adjustments to the open-ended questions in the second section of the climate survey tool. We changed the open-ended questions and framed them carefully to ensure positive responses. We did the same for the appreciative inquiry and behavioral event interview questions. We had to test those questions to be sure that they got at the positive, successful examples. We did not want to ask leading questions that would bias the responses. We wanted the responses to be as truthful as possible.

Crafting the interview questions was difficult because most individuals are comfortable with the expert model. For example some interviewees wanted to say what they *thought* leadership should be. They wanted to report what expert leaders do. We had to reframe the questions to elicit the telling of *actual* behaviors and the thoughts that led to them. Also, we had to explain our behavioral model to our contributors. We had to say, "Look, we are not looking for examples of what you believe leadership should be. Just report the stories you heard in the interviews." Those who were telling the stories and those conveying them to the reader, had to remain true to that approach.

Each set of interviews yielded hundreds of pages of transcripts, and from those pages, we needed to decide what stories were exemplars and therefore worthy of imitation. They were all great stories. Which ones should we use in the book? That is where the assessment tools and the data gathered from the behavioral event interviews came into play. We looked at the results of the assessments and identified trends and patterns. Those trends and patterns painted the picture of which stories we would pull out. Stories that supported the assessments would be the construct that drove the chapter.

The behavioral event interviews were coded. We used thematic coding to help get at the competencies. After we had the case examples, we then came up with a cluster of themes that represented the essence of the organization. We then recoded all of the stories by those organizational themes. It was a five-, six-, seven-, eight-step process of actually writing the chapter.

We grouped the stories within those themes. Some of the stories represent cross-cutting themes for all organizations, and some were very unique to each masterpiece organization. These themes became the topic headings that appear in the organizational case study chapters. These headings are not meant to be prescriptive in nature; they are simply a way to organize the stories. In fact, some of the best stories fit in more than one category.

It was interesting to watch this process emerge within the masterpiece organizations. Although the contributors were collecting stories through appreciative inquiry, they did not know the results of the assessments, nor did they know the content of the behavioral event interviews and the competencies uncovered in those interviews. Likewise, as we coded the Behavioral Event Interviews and scored the assessments, we had no idea what stories the contributors were collecting. It was amazing to later see how the stories supported the data and vice versa.

As we went through this process, we were doing our own exploration around storytelling. In particular, we gravitated toward Stephen Denning's (2000) works around the "springboard" story. We knew that the stories uncovered were great exemplars, but how would we select from so many? How would we decide what part of each story was relevant for our masterpiece book? The theory behind the springboard story helped us to identify each particular story we captured. Now we knew just what pieces of the story needed to be told to make it a valuable tool. That became part of the training and knowledge sharing we conducted with our contributors.

MASTERPIECE SUMMIT

About nine months after we began the pilot, our contributors had completed their appreciative inquiry interviews, and we were writing our first drafts. We held a summit that brought all of the contributors and the leaders of the organizations together for a day and a half of sharing, celebrating, and exploring next steps. This gathering provided a testing ground to evaluate the impact of the stories we uncovered.

As we organized the summit event we selected stories that had been uncovered at each organization to share with all of the participants. The night before and the morning of the summit, we were very anxious about sharing these stories. How would they come across? What impact, if any, would they have?

As soon as we shared the first story, we knew that the entire project would be well received. The stories were no longer just poignant and thought provoking: They were exemplars that moved even the successful leaders who inspired them. When we posed the question "what is the difference between a great work of art and a masterpiece," there was dead silence in the room. Everybody was listening, suddenly more alert and anxious to hear the answer. When we revealed the answer—"passion"—everybody became fully engaged and started taking notes. At that point, we knew we were going to have an impact for the rest of the day.

One participant summarized, "All of us in healthcare are doing great works of art. We all provide the same services. It is those of us who have *passion* about our work who are the ones who are actually creating masterpieces in healthcare." It was a profound statement!

The stories we shared at the summit came alive and brought these already successful leaders to a higher level of passion, excitement, and drive to perpetuate their success. It stimulated their table discussions about challenges, successes, and sustainability around their hopes and dreams for the future. It was quite powerful and also validated the value of the stories that we had uncovered. We knew that we could then solidify our process and work with the contributors to complete their chapters.

Reference

Denning, S. (2000). *The springboard: How storytelling ignites action in knowledge-era organizations.* Boston: Butterworth-Heinemann.

CHAPTER 2

Research Methods

Although we used the philosophies of artists (da Vinci and Karsh) to guide us in our journey to uncover leadership masterpieces and chose the art of storytelling to present our excavations, our research is steeply based in behavioral science. This chapter describes our scientific approach to gathering the data.

HEALTHCARE CAUSAL FLOW LEADERSHIP MODEL

We used the Healthcare Causal Flow Leadership Model (based on the initial research of David McClelland and colleagues at the Harvard Business School and the subsequent work of others in the field of behavioral sciences) to guide our data collection. "Their collective research, ongoing since the 1950s, indicates that successful leadership competencies and leadership styles produce a motivating environment or healthcare climate which arouse employee motivation to work well, and predict the desired organizational outcomes: exceptional patient satisfaction and financial performance" (Spencer, Pelote, & Seymour, 1998).

Figure 2-1 depicts the Healthcare Causal Flow Leadership Model as a series of seven variables, including three independent healthcare leadership variables, three patient moderator variables, and one dependent healthcare outcome variable linked in a causal flow. The model suggests the following:

- The effects of leadership directly influence healthcare climate.
- High healthcare climate is likely to have a positive influence on staff–patient encounters that in turn predict patient satisfaction and clinical outcomes.

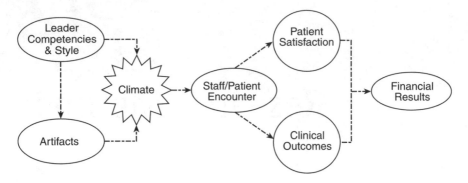

FIGURE 2-1   Healthcare Causal Flow Leadership Model. Published by the editor at UMMC, adapted from the UMMC-Hay McBer Causal Leadership Model, 1998.

- Artifacts positively impact climate and also support leader competencies and style.

Many healthcare leaders tend to focus their attention and energy on financial results, clinical outcomes, and patient satisfaction, which are the core of healthcare. In our causal flow model, we posit that these represent dependent variables. The independent variables that impact the dependent variables in a causal-flow relationship are leader competencies and style, resources or artifacts, and healthcare climate. Collectively, these variables impact the staff–patient encounters and the remaining dependent variables. We use this Healthcare Causal Flow Leadership Model to frame the findings and conclusions of our research.

BEHAVIORAL COMPETENCIES

A behavioral competency is a pattern of behavior that is defined in terms of a thought–action sequence. The competency dictionary that we use is a classification of those behaviors grouped according to the nature of the behaviors. Table 2-1 lists 21 competencies grouped into four categories. A general definition follows each of those competencies.

Each leadership competency is further broken down into nine levels that represent specific behaviors described in terms of a specific thought–action sequence. Table 2-2 depicts the specific behavior levels in the leading others competency, a general competency in the power and influence category.

Table 2-1   Competency Groupings and Definitions

Self-Management	1	Achievement motivation	Looks to make things systematically better.
	2	Concern for order	Pays attention to details and organizes them.
	3	Flexibility	Changes behaviors and/or actions.
	4	Integrity	Does the "right" thing based on espoused values.
	5	Self-confidence	Takes on risky assignments or confronts those in power.
	6	Self-control	Controls strong emotions, especially negative emotions and/or anger.
Power and Influence	7	Change leadership	Builds commitment in others to move toward the future.
	8	Developing others	Looks to develop skills and behaviors of others.
	9	Clear direction	Sets standards for behavior and performance and holds people accountable.
	10	Impact and influence	Develops and uses strategies and tactics to impact or influence others.
	11	Leading others	Motivates groups of people to achieve results.
	12	Organizational awareness	Recognizes the realities of organizational politics and structure.
	13	Relationship building	Builds professional relationships either at work or outside of the workplace.
Logic and Reasoning	14	Analytical thinking	Understands and applies cause and effect relationships.
	15	Conceptual thinking	Matches patterns and assembles varied pieces into a coherent whole.
	16	Creative thinking	Uses alternative and innovative thinking in developing solutions.
	17	Future thinking	Thinks ahead to act on future needs or prevent problems.
	18	Information seeking	Gathers information for self and/or others.
Helping and Caring	19	Customer service focus	Acts on behalf of the person being served.
	20	Inquiry	Seeks to understand what others are saying, feeling, and thinking.
	21	Teamwork and cooperation	Looks to achieve results as a team and genuinely respects other team members.

Adapted from Spencer, L., & Spencer, S. (1993). *Competency at work: Models for superior performance.* NY: Wiley.

Table 2-2   Behavioral Competency Level Descriptions

Leading Others

Motivates groups of people to achieve results

Level	Description
-1	Undermines subordinate efforts.
0	Focuses on completing own tasks.
1	Makes sure the group has all the necessary information. Explains the reasons for a decision.
2	Makes sure the practical and emotional needs of the group are met.
3	Makes a personal effort to treat all group members fairly.
4	Clearly articulates the links between performance and customer expectations.
5	Recognizes and rewards performance.
6	Ensures that others buy into leader's mission, goals, agenda, tone, and policy.
7	Communicates a compelling vision that generates excitement, enthusiasm, and commitment.

DATA COLLECTION

Data were collected using four types of assessment instruments: Behavioral Event Interviews (BEI), Appreciative Inquiry (AI) interviews, the Healthcare Leadership Inventory, and the Healthcare Organizational Climate Survey. The BEI and the Leadership Inventory were used to gather leadership competency data. Leadership style data were gathered from the Healthcare Leadership Inventory. Healthcare climate data were gathered from a separate assessment. Each of these assessments is described in this chapter.

Table 2-3 lists the individuals and groups from each of the organizations targeted to participate in the data collection. It also shows which interview and assessment types were used.

Interviews

BEIs

The BEI is a structured process in which we asked the leaders to describe critical, work-related incidents that they actively participated in. We

Table 2-3   Summary of Data Collection Instruments and Participants

Participant	Interviews		Assessments	
	BEI	AI	Healthcare Leadership Inventory	Climate Survey Tool
CEO/president/academic chair	X	X	X	
Senior leadership individual	X	X	X	
Senior leader group	X	X	X	
Manager(s), focus area	X	X	X	X
Individual staff member		X		X
Staff, focus area focus group (7 to 9 participants)		X		X
Patient from study area individual		X		
Patients from study area focus group (7 to 9 participants)		X		
Individual stakeholder				
Stakeholders focus group (7 to 9 participants)		X		

asked for these critical incidents to be expressed in short-story detail. In an open-ended, question-and-answer format, we asked the following questions: "What led up to the situation?" "Who was involved?" "What did you think about, feel, or want to have happen in the situation." "What did you do?" "What was the outcome?"

The interviews were recorded and transcribed. We used the information from the transcriptions in two ways: (1) as exemplar stories that are part of the masterpiece chapters and (2) as thought–action–sequence data that were coded as evidence of the leadership competencies.

We used the information from the BEI transcripts to code for the competencies spontaneously described by the interviewees. Each behavior or thought–action sequence elicited in the interview was matched to a specific behavior in the competency dictionary (see Tables 2-1 and 2-2 for sample competency dictionary pages). For example, if the interviewee stated, "I wanted to improve our check-in process," we translated this response to *achievement motivation* (a desire to do better). If the interviewee mentioned taking time to listen to a patient's concern about surgery, we translated this response to *customer-service focus* (a desire to meet underlying needs of the patient). If the interviewee said, "So I surveyed a sample of our patients about what we could do better," we translated this response to *information seeking* (takes action to gather information for self and others).

We conducted 52 BEIs within the nine organizations featured in this book. From those 52 interviews, we coded 947 events, which translates to 18 significant events per hour in which the leaders positively impacted the healthcare climate.

AI Interviews

The exemplar stories that comprise a large part of the masterpiece chapters were extracted from the BEIs and also from the AI interviews that our contributors conducted. We used the work of David L. Cooperrider and Diana Whitney as a guide for the appreciative exploration. In their book *A Positive Revolution in Change: Appreciative Inquiry*, Cooperrider and Whitney (2005), state the following:

> Appreciative inquiry is about the co-evolutionary search for the best in people, their organizations, and the relevant world around them. In its broadest focus, it involves systematic discovery of what gives "life" to a living system when it is most alive, most effective, and most constructively capable in economic, ecological, and human terms.
>
> AI involves, in a central way, the art and practice of asking questions that strengthen a system's capacity to apprehend, anticipate, and heighten positive potential. It centrally involves the mobilization of inquiry through the crafting of the "unconditional positive question" often-involving hundreds or sometimes thousands of people. In AI the arduous task of intervention gives way to the speed of imagination and innovation; instead of negation, criticism, and spiraling diagnosis, there is discovery, dream, and design.

Interview Totals

In both the BEI and AI interviews, we were looking to uncover the underlying thoughts, actions, hopes, and dreams from a positive perspective. We were careful not to put our own mental models into people's minds. We wanted to allow individuals to be truthful as they were telling their stories. Each time we heard these stories through the interviews or read

Table 2-4   Interview Participants

List of Participants	
Corporate CEOs	Nurses
CEOs	Medical residents
Executive leadership	Ancillary and support staff
Vice-presidents	Patients and residents
Directors	Family members
Managers	Community members
Physicians	

Number of BEIs	52
Number of AIs	95
Individual AI interviews	54
Focus group AI interviews	41
Total number of individuals interviewed	324
BEI hours	54 hours
AI interview hours	116 hours

the transcripts of those interviews or felt the reaction of others when we shared the stories, it unveiled another layer of "wow."

BEI and AI interviews were conducted at the executive leadership level of the organization and also at the director and manager level of the focus area. AI interviews were also conducted with the staff, stakeholders, and patients within the focus area of each organization. The AI interviews consisted of both individual and focus groups. These interviews were also recorded and transcribed so that the stories and exemplars from these interviews could be combined with the stories from the BEIs to form the basis of the masterpiece chapters.

Table 2-4 lists the numbers of interviews conducted.

Healthcare Leadership Inventory

The healthcare leadership inventory identified leadership strengths, competencies, and style (see Table 2-4 for a list of those who completed the healthcare leadership inventory assessment). This self-assessment questionnaire took approximately 15 to 20 minutes to complete. Leaders selected the competencies and style that they felt were most reflective of their leadership practices. The assessment that we used consisted of 45 questions. The questionnaire consisted of two sections. Section 1 identified leadership competencies, and Section 2 identified leadership style.

Leadership Competencies

The section of the healthcare leadership inventory pertaining to leadership competencies contained questions crafted from the competency behavior levels in the competency dictionary. A competency is "what outstanding performers do more often, in more situations, with better results, than average performers" (Spencer & Spencer, 1993). In general terms, competencies can be thought of as a series of knowledge, skills, and behavioral attributes. Spencer, in *Competence at Work*, defined competencies as "an underlying characteristic of an individual which is causally related to effective or superior (one standard deviation above the mean) performance in a job" (Spencer & Spencer).

Leadership competencies should also be thought of as underlying attributes or patterns of behavior required to achieve superior performance in a work setting. It is what successful leaders do more often to achieve superior results (Spencer, Pelote, & Seymour, 1998). The leader's self-assessment of the behavioral competencies were compared with the actual evidence of this behavior elicited from the coded BEIs.

Leadership Style

Leadership style is the way in which a leader relates to staff and colleagues. Table 2-5 describes six leadership styles derived from research conducted by the editors while at Value Added Performance in collaboration with

Table 2-5   Leadership Styles That Predict Organizational Climate

Leadership Style	Definition of Leadership Style
Affiliative	Concern for people leader
Authoritative	Expert leader
Coaching	Developing others leader
Coercive	"Do it or else" leader
Democratic	Involve others leader
Pacesetting	"Do it myself" leader

Source: Adapted from editors' presentation, ASTD, 1992.

Hay/McBer and the American Society for Training and Development. According to this research, any one or all of the styles described in Table 2-5 are effective, depending on the demands of the situation, the employees' skill level and needs, and the resources available (Pelote, DeWitt, & Dreyfus, 1992).

We used the data collected from the leadership style self assessment in two ways: (1) to help us select which stories were examples of the leadership styles in action within the organizations and (2) to represent the collective styles of leadership in the masterpiece organizations as they fit into the Healthcare Leadership Causal Flow Model.

Healthcare Climate Survey

The healthcare climate survey consists of two sections. The first section contains 18 multiple-choice questions. The second section consists of four open-ended questions. It was distributed to all employees within the focus area. "Healthcare climate can be thought of as a pervasive atmosphere or environment that influences all organization members. Positive climate arouses employee motivation to do jobs well and to improve outcomes continuously for patients" (Spencer, Pelote, & Seymour, 1998).

We break healthcare climate into six distinct dimensions. Each one of these dimensions provides measures of how energizing and motivating the work environment is for employees. Table 2-6 describes the six dimensions of the healthcare climate.

Table 2-6   Six Dimensions of the Healthcare Climate

Dimension	Description
Accountability and responsibility	Leadership treats employees fairly and follows through on commitments
Innovative and flexible processes and structures	Resources are available to do the work and there is input for making improvements.
Clarity	Purpose, goals, and procedures are clear
Reward and recognition	Recognition is directly related to levels of performance and expectations
Pride and expectations	There is pride in the clinical outcomes and patient satisfaction, meaningful work, and a safe work environment.
Teamwork and cooperation	Employees work cooperatively and trust and support each other

Source: Adapted from editors' presentation, ASTD, 1992.

The Healthcare Climate Survey was completed by employees from eight of the nine organizations featured in this text. It explained the impact of the leadership behaviors and style we uncovered as they relate to the Healthcare Leadership Causal Flow Model.

References

Spencer, L., Pelote, V., & Seymour, P. (1998). A Causal Model and Research Paradigm for Physicians as Leaders of Change. *New Medicine, Vol. 2*, 57-64.

Pelote, V., DeWitt, F., and Dreyfus, C. (1992). *Measuring management's impact upon total quality*. Annual Meeting of the American Society for Training and Development. New Orleans, Louisiana.

Cooperrider, D., & Whitney, D. (2005). *Appreciative inquiry: A positive revolution in change*. San Francisco: Berrett-Koehler Publishers.

Spencer, L., & Spencer, S. (1993). *Competency at work: Models for superior performance*. NY: Wiley.

CHAPTER 3

Data Analysis

In Chapter 2 we talked about the Healthcare Causal Flow Leadership Model and the various assessment tools that we used to collect data that fit within the model. We introduced our hypothesis about the impact that leadership has in creating a motivating environment for employees. In this chapter, we share some of the high-level results from the data collection and the conclusions that we have drawn from the data.

BEHAVIORAL EVENT INTERVIEWS ANALYSIS

From the 52 behavioral event interviews (BEIs) we conducted, the codable events (described in Chapter 2) are summarized in Figure 3-1. These BEIs were conducted within a cross-section of the leadership from each of the nine masterpiece organizations. During these interviews, the leaders shared many stories or events that were important and critical to their success. The interviews were recorded and transcribed. From these interviews, we extracted 947 instances of leadership behaviors that fell within 21 competency behaviors.

We divided those results into four categories: most, moderate, some, and very little. Figure 3-1 clearly shows where masterpiece leaders spend their time. When considering how masterpiece leaders prioritize their time, look at the competencies that the leaders focus on both the most and the least.

These data reveal that the masterpiece leaders spend most of their time on behaviors that allow them to engage and nurture staff, reward and recognize staff, and provide the resources to continuously improve.

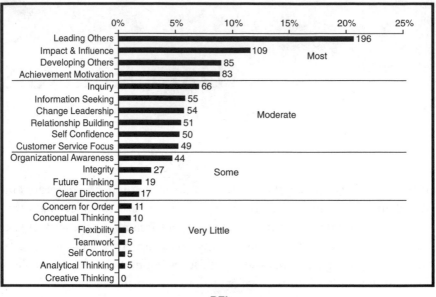

Where Masterpiece Leaders Spend Their Time

BEI
Codable Events
N = 947

FIGURE 3-1   Where Masterpiece Leaders Spend Their Time

BEI Conclusion 1

Masterpiece leaders spend most of their time leading others.

We define leading others as motivating staff members to achieve desired results by recognizing, rewarding, and engaging them. Thus, what do these leaders think about? Their foremost thought is this: "How do I motivate my staff?" These types of thoughts lead to the behaviors of engaging, rewarding, and recognizing others. Masterpiece leaders are successful because they constantly think about motivating their staff and finding ways to provide meaningful rewards and recognition.

Leading others also has to do with day-to-day leadership. It's not just "all right we need to fix this. Let's engage the staff. Let's motivate them." The behaviors associated with leading others are not just for special occasions. Every day the leaders are constantly engaging, rewarding, and recognizing their staff members.

BEI Conclusion 2

Masterpiece leaders are constantly thinking about ways to have a positive impact by persuading others.

The second competency where leaders spend most of their time is impact and influence, which has to do with powerful persuasion. Masterpiece leaders think about how they can get others to do what is important for their organization, their staff, and their patients. Although some may be inclined to interpret this as persuading people for their own personal benefit or manipulating others, we interpret this behavior as trying to help people move toward a greater good.

BEI Conclusion 3

Masterpiece leaders spend considerable time thinking about the short- and long-term professional growth of their staff.

The third competency where masterpiece leaders spend most of their time is developing others. They are genuinely concerned about the professional development of their staff members—not just about getting their own idea across. They view themselves as a leader–educator, not as a leader–expert. The leader–expert has knowledge that he or she feels the need to impart to people because of his or her expertise. The leader–educator is concerned with sharing knowledge. He or she is concerned about sharing this knowledge in a way that enables people's growth and he or she is really good at assessing staff's strengths and weaknesses and then providing opportunities for success. The leader–educator provides assignments so that their staff members can continually learn and improve.

BEI Conclusion 4

Masterpiece leaders relentlessly focus on what is most important and continuously find ways to make things better.

The fourth competency in which masterpiece leaders spend most of their time is achievement motivation. These leaders continuously think about ways to make things better and also provide the resources to support improvements. They are not just preaching it or doing it all themselves; instead, they are enabling the culture and the staff to improve continuously. This applies when things are going well as well as when things are not going well. It applies to day-to day operations in addition to when there is a crisis.

BEI Conclusion 5

Masterpiece leaders spend 8% (a very small amount) of their time on the seven competencies: creative, analytical, and conceptual thinking; self-control, flexibility, teamwork, and concern for order.

The data in Figure 3-1 show that leaders spend less time on the behaviors that involve fixing day-to-day problems. They trust and rely on their employees to handle the day to day issues.

LEADERSHIP STYLE ANALYSIS

The masterpiece leaders completed a multiple-choice self-assessment on their leadership style (see Chapter 2). The data gathered concluded that masterpiece leaders view their role as having a positive impact by engaging their staff, improving processes, creating the future, and coaching. Their collective preferred leadership style is to engage and coach their staff. They are comfortable with the uncertainty that comes with engaging staff. Their backup styles balance this leadership style. When required, they also show a genuine concern for the people and use their expertise to direct others.

As shown in Figure 3-2, masterpiece leaders see themselves as relying on two dominant or preferred styles. These styles are democratic (77%) and coaching (60%). The two styles that they use as back up are affiliative

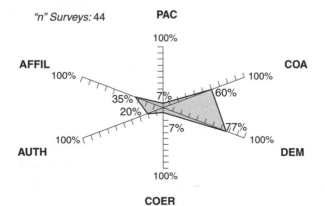

FIGURE 3-2   Masterpiece leaders self-assessment of their leadership style.

(35%) and authoritative (20%). These leaders do not see themselves as pacesetting (doing the work themselves) or coercive (threatening others to do the work).

Dominant Leadership Styles

The following are descriptions for the leadership styles that the masterpiece leaders prefer.

Democratic

Democratic leaders ask staff members for their thoughts and opinions. They involve them in the decision-making process. They consistently round and seek out suggestions for making improvements and routinely hold all-staff meetings. They share patient satisfaction results with staff and engage staff in making improvements.

Coaching

Coaching leaders are concerned about their staff's professional and personal development. They coach them on two levels. One level involves helping them with, for example, the content of their presentations and dealing with their peers and subordinates. On another level, that leader helps that same employee explore career paths and the importance of, for example, public speaking.

Backup Leadership Styles

Although masterpiece leaders prefer to engage or coach their staff, there may be times when they realize that a different style is appropriate for the situation. The affiliative or authoritative style may be needed. For instance, if the work is not getting done and a deadline is looming, then these leaders would use an authoritative style by saying this: "This is where we're going. This is what we need to do, and this is when we need to do it by." Their direction would be very clear. They would explain what needed to be accomplished, and they would set very clear expectations.

The following descriptions describe the affiliative and authoritative styles that our masterpiece leaders use as their backup style approach to leading.

Affiliative

Affiliative leaders are genuinely concerned for people and their well-being. These leaders are concerned about the individual and their family. They are concerned with how their staff is balancing work and home life.

Authoritative

Authoritative leaders use their expertise as the foundation for sharing with others. This may sound negative. Some may see this type of leadership style as similar to coercive or confuse it with the word authoritarian. An enormous difference exists between coercive and authoritative. Coercive leaders threaten others. Leaders who use an authoritative style are very explicit in their expectations. They are extremely clear about the tasks at hand. These leaders also use data to add clarity and allow their staff to understand the rationale or deeper meaning behind the expectations.

Seldom-Used Leadership Styles

Masterpiece leaders do not use pacesetting and coercive styles. When you read the exemplar chapters, you will see very little or no evidence of either of these styles. Here is a description of those unused styles.

Pacesetting

Pacesetting leaders do the work themselves. They feel that if they want something done right, they have to do it themselves. They also believe that no one can do it better than they can.

Coercive

Coercive leaders lead by threatening others to get the work done. Their preference is to give ultimatums. Coercive leaders may also resort to bullying.

CLIMATE SURVEY ANALYSIS

In Chapter 2, we described the Healthcare Climate Survey Tool. This was a paper and pencil survey distributed to the staff within the focus area in eight of the nine masterpiece organizations. We posited that in the Healthcare Causal Flow Model the climate is directly impacted by leadership competencies and style. We measured six dimensions of healthcare climate in our survey. These dimensions are listed in Figure 3-3.

FIGURE 3-3   Six Dimensions of the Healthcare Climate

Dimension	Description
Accountability and responsibility	Leadership treats employees fairly and follows through on commitments
Innovative and flexible processes and structures	Resources are available to do the work and there is input for making improvements.
Clarity	Purpose, goals, and procedures are clear
Reward and recognition	Recognition is directly related to levels of performance and expectations
Pride and expectations	There is pride in the clinical outcomes and patient satisfaction, meaningful work, and a safe work environment.
Teamwork and cooperation	Employees work cooperatively and trust and support each other

Source: Adapted from editors' presentation, ASTD, 1992.

The results from our data collection are very similar to previous research that the editors conducted in a study published by the American Society for Training and Development. In discussing this research, Steve Kelner noted in the *Center for Quality & Management Journal* that "the study findings showed that the positive organizational climate created by successful TQM managers was significantly higher than those created by the unsuccessful ones. Normed against a database of more than 2,000 managers worldwide, the summary measure of climate was more than 30 percentile points higher for the best than the rest" (Kelner, 1998).

The Healthcare Climate Survey results displayed in Figure 3-4 compare masterpiece organizational scores against other healthcare organizations. The comparison scores are displayed by using a percentile ranking. The 50th percentile is the average climate score. Staff performance is generally enhanced when the overall climate is high (above 60%).

The overall climate for the masterpiece organizations is very high. It is 30 percentile points higher than the average healthcare organization. Although our sample size is small, the results compare favorably with previous research. There is also evidence of a high climate in the supporting stories and comments that are in the following chapters.

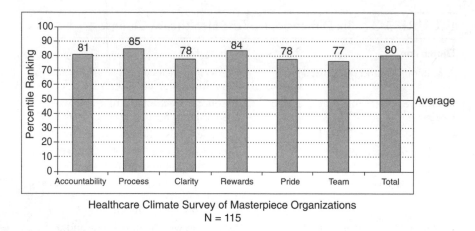

FIGURE 3-4   Masterpiece Focus Area Climate Survey Results

The two highest climate dimensions within the masterpiece organizations are process and rewards. Given that leading others and achievement motivation are two of the competencies where leaders spend most of their time and the two dominant leadership styles are democratic and coaching, it is not surprising that staff members feel strongly that they have the resources to do their work, they have input into making things better, and report being recognized for the work that they do.

CONCLUSIONS

Masterpiece leaders have created systems that have a positive impact in holding people accountable by engaging staff, following through on commitments, and being actively involved with activities such as rounding. They have coached the staff so that their performance has improved. It is apparent that by creating a nurturing, open, and engaging leadership style that masterpiece leaders have also created an environment where staff members work closely together as a team where they trust and respect each other. These organizations also present a clear purpose that the staff can identify with. It is not the mission statement that motivates staff; instead, it is the higher calling that is constantly communicated by leadership to staff. Staff members are deeply connected with each other, to their work, to their leaders, and to the mission of their organizations. Our stories will demonstrate the incredible pride staff members have in working at these organizations.

Reference

Kelner, S. P. (1999). Organizational climate and TQM. *Journal for the Center for Quality Management, 7*(1).

CHAPTER 4

How to Read the Stories

STORY SELECTION

Our mission was to illustrate in story form 1) key leadership behaviors, 2) staff conduct that resulted from the leadership behaviors, and 3) outcomes of these behaviors. We present those through the voices of the individuals we interviewed. We believe stories are a powerful way to present these complex ideas. All of us have heard that "a picture paints a thousand words." We posit "a story paints a thousand pictures."

Success that seems to come easy for some does not happen by chance. The individual and collective stories we present embody those patterns of behavior that are worthy of imitation. After hearing interviews and rereading transcripts of those interviews, we experienced the power of the pure stories. Those words made us say "wow" and think deeply about their impact. We did not want to alter those stories in a way that would limit the endless messages that the stories might send to others. In an effort to recreate the original thought-provoking stories, we quoted the words of the transcripts with very little paraphrasing.

In keeping with Stephen Denning's work *The Springboard: How Storytelling Ignites Action in Knowledge-Era Organizations*, we considered how we might transmit concepts, attitudes, and skills that are barely understood. How could we explain to a group that what they have done for the past years had to be discarded and abandoned? By telling a story.

In his work, Denning tells us that a story can communicate a new idea quickly, easily, and naturally. We don't have to be taught how to do this. We do it naturally and find it relaxing and energizing. Even when sleeping we dream in stories. Our challenge was to include just enough to spark a new story in the mind of the reader.

Another variable that we considered when we selected our stories was the results of our assessment tools. We needed to think about the leadership styles and behavioral competencies that we extracted from our research. The stories that were examples of these data needed to be included.

We were left with a collection of stories and statements that had no particular rhyme or reason. We needed to make sense of them—organize them somehow. The solution was to insert topic headings to help the reader to recognize and zero in on topics of interest. So, we created topic headings in each of the masterpiece chapters. They are not meant to interpret or analyze the stories but simply frame the stories.

The last step in the writing process was editing the stories. We wanted the reader to have the same gut response to the stories as we had when listening to the interviews. The closer we kept to the dialogue, the better the message would ring true. Although we were very careful to write the stories as they were told, we could not always include the words from the transcript verbatim. We needed to change the spoken word into written and did some slight paraphrasing to make the story clear.

Because the goal of our masterpiece is not to recognize a particular person but to illustrate the successful behavior, we have let some stories stand on their own. When you read the stories, you may not know who is speaking, but you will understand the behavior. We hope that this will inspire you to imitate the behaviors and create your own stories.

THE FOCUS AREA

Our research included data collection from the executive leadership in each of the organizations. In addition, we wanted to understand the impact of that leadership and highlight the impact it had through the voices of the staff, patients, stakeholders, and members of the community. To accomplish this, we identified a focus area or department that was representative of the organization. This selected focus area isolated a particular unit, department, or area that fell under the umbrella of the executive leadership.

The exemplar stories you are about to read include the recollections of the executive leadership and a sampling of individuals from the focus area.

THE VOICES

Each of the organizations profiled in this book has received numerous accolades and awards. Although we invited them to be part of this book because of those accomplishments, we chose not to describe all the phases of their journey or fully recognize those involved in their success. Instead, we focus on those stories that depict the leadership behaviors, stories from staff members and stakeholders that result from these leadership behaviors, and the impact that these behaviors have on patients.

The stories are presented without introduction, interpretation, assumptions, or analysis. You may read several versions of the same story. In some cases, the role of the speaker will be apparent; in others, it will not. In all cases, the motivation of the behavior, the impact, and the result will be apparent. Enjoy.

Table 5-1 Organizational Demographics

Organization	Clinton Hospital
Location	Clinton, MA
Setting	Rural
Communities served	Suburban and rural
Type of organization	Community hospital
Number of beds	41
Number of Full Time Equivalents (FTEs)	176
Scope of service	Full-service hospital offering a variety of outpatient and inpatient services
Focus area	Emergency department
Focus number served	Services approximately 11,000 patients per year from the local surrounding communities
Focus area Best practices and awards	2006 Press Ganey Summit Award

CHAPTER 5

The Pilot

Clinton Hospital is a full-service community hospital located in Clinton, Massachusetts. Their emergency department—our focus area—services approximately 12,000 patients per year from the local surrounding communities.

Clinton Hospital was gracious in allowing us to use their facility as a pilot for our masterpiece project. We needed to test our interview questions, instructions for completing assessments, and time commitment and involvement. We wanted a local organization that we could partner with and one that had also met the criteria for success. As members of the local community, we had heard positive stories about the excellent care received at Clinton Hospital. We knew also that their overall patient satisfaction scores were high, especially in their emergency department. In talking with their CEO, we learned that Clinton Hospital used Press Ganey for measuring patient satisfaction in their emergency department. She shared with us that when compared with other Massachusetts Hospitals, the Clinton Hospital Emergency Department had ranked in the 93rd to 95th percentile for overall satisfaction with care.

After meeting with the executive team, we identified an extensive list of individuals to interview. We met with all members of the executive team, physician and nursing leadership in the emergency department, staff, patients, and members of the community. The stories we uncovered were equally as impressive as the organizations featured in this book. We would be remiss if we did not share their stories of success.

CLINTON HOSPITAL

Work—Life Balance

At Clinton Hospital, employees are able to maintain a balance between life and work. This is something that you don't find frequently in health care. I think that's what other people struggle with in finding leaders in health care.

Everybody's home life is different, but if things aren't working at home, they are not going to be working in that ER. Bottom line—it's a rare bird that can separate home and be 100% at work.

A key thing is to always keep in mind the staff's personal lives. My goal is to help them get their schedules so that it works for their home life. If you have somebody who has kids that play football and are really big into football, try to give them all of the game days off. Football season is short. The scheduling takes a little bit of effort, but if you give them that kind of attention it helps them maintain that balance.

If you say, "How did the game go last week?" That helps 600%. It helps them want to be at work. If they have the time off they need, then they enjoy coming to work. When they want to be at work they give better care. If they can't wait to get out of work, then they're not committed. If you show them fairness and understanding in their personal needs and personal life, they will "pick up an extra day, or stay a little longer than their shift."

One of my staff had a baby. We had a whole discussion about childcare issues. She thought she would have to leave. "You know what?" I said. "We need to see how we can work your time and your schedule." She works 12-hour shifts, so I put her on a shorter day and gave her some benefit time. We split her schedule up. I never put her 2 days in row, so that if she were up with the baby at night she would have enough time to rest. If there was a day when I had extra staff, I gave her the choice of having the day off.

A staff member states, "We all have personal things going on in our own lives, and in the seven years I have been here, I've only missed one personal event. When issues come up or family members are ill, they help us. This place has really been tremendous in that respect—looking out for each other."

One of our co-workers lost a husband and was scheduled to work on Christmas. She posted a note asking whether anybody could volunteer just a few hours so that she could be with her kids. Everyone of us took a few hours that Christmas Day to come in so she could be home with her family.

A typical comment of one of the nurses is this: "It's my job, and it is not just my job, I love coming in. I love working and I love taking care of the patients and I love who I'm working with. If I get called in to work, I know it's for a good reason. I'm not angry that I got called in. That's my job."

Patients First

One of her things is total, total, total: The patients come first—the patient comes first. Our manager has drummed that into us for so many years that we are getting kind of sick of it, but she does have a point.

In everything we do, we have to make sure the patient is at the center. That's what our being is. That's what we're here for. I have to stay focused on that because if in my job I'm not focused on that, chances are other people are not going to be.

If we don't have patients, we don't exist. So somehow we have to make sure that we are an essential service in the community.

You want to go home at the end of the day and believe that any patient that comes through your doors has received good care. I felt that I could leave my staff comfortably knowing that patients were going to get what they needed.

Nobody is sitting at the nurse's station when there are patients in the rooms. That's the first thing. I observe that all of the time. The staff has their little "war stories" about how that pays off. One nurse had a patient come in the other day who was complaining of severe arm pain. The nurse took the patient right from the door right into the trauma room and began treating her appropriately. She put the IV in, got the oxygen on, medicated her, and never left the room. The patient arrested right in front of her within 10 minutes of arrival. That nurse felt great satisfaction in the fact that she could not have done more. There was nothing that could have happened differently. She didn't leave her in the waiting room thinking she would "get to her in a little while" or "we'll wait for the labs." The staff gets satisfaction in knowing when they go back and look at things that they couldn't have done it differently. Those are the good points.

I talk about patient satisfaction all of the time. "Why are they waiting over there? Did you go talk to them? What's their next step?" I talk to them all the time about that. I will tell you that staff will give me the "busy" story. I tell them, "Busy is better. If you weren't busy, you wouldn't have a reason to have to go back to anybody because there would be nobody to go back to. There would be nobody waiting. So we wouldn't even be having this conversation, and your job security would be in the toilet. So, busy is not a good reason."

I've had nurses who have been sick in other emergency departments, and they come back to the table and say, "I know what she's talking about. I was in such and such—do you know that that damn nurse walked by me 68 times and didn't say one word to me?"

We walk by these people a lot. We should be probably saying something to them. "The doctor's seeing two more people and then he should be with you," or "we're waiting for the lab to turn around your lab work" or whatever. That helps to reinforce the whole—"you just have to walk in those shoes for a little while." That's the whole management style, too. If you walk in their shoes, get down and work in that emergency department, for two hours or an hour every day, you get to understand what they're saying. You get to appreciate that.

I was working one night, and we had a lady who was very confused. She couldn't get A and B together and hadn't really been like that previously. I went to get the restraint so that she wouldn't fall out of the bed.

The nurse who was on that day said, "You know what? Let's call her son to come see her. Maybe he can settle her in so that we won't need to restrain her."

I said, "That's a cool idea." So she called the son, and indeed, the son came in and sat with her for an hour or two. She settled down, and we never put the restraint on.

I had a patient a couple of years ago when I was new to the ER. The patient and his family wanted to go elsewhere for a second opinion. I encouraged them to go even though I wasn't sure I should. Surprisingly, my boss supported me. She told the patient, "If you want to be transferred to get a second opinion, that is your right and your privilege." Later, that family contacted me and thanked me profusely. I thought that was just unbelievable that I was able, with my boss's approval, to do that.

I value the trust that my patients put in me. I treasure that. They are so appreciative that I am able to draw blood without hurting them. It just gives me the sense that I've made a difference in their life, especially if they hate needles and are afraid of them.

As the secretary, I get to observe a lot. I get to see patients when they come in, and I talk to their families. I've seen the nurses work on the patients and watch them put all of their efforts into these patients as if they were their own family members. The families come out and tell me that they had a wonderful experience and that they want to tell someone. "Who can I tell about the excellent staff here? I hope you guys are here forever." That is one of the high points of my job.

I think there needs to be balance in health care in general. You can have all of the technology that you want, but if you don't have someone holding the hands of a patient, you still don't have the whole picture. I think that everybody in healthcare should be looking for that balance and trying to make sure that they deliver both to our patients. You can do that here.

Underlying Needs of Patients

The police brought in a female patient with a psychiatric problem. The ER was full at the time. I remember putting her in the quiet room while the staff was busy trying to make room someplace else. I wanted to get her out of the hall so that she wasn't the center of attention. I was thinking, "This poor girl—I don't want everybody to see her in the hall." So, my first thought was to get her some privacy, some safety, and then my second thought was how am I going to get this woman the care she needs right now.

I happened to mention that I wanted the police to go to her home to be sure her children were safe. If there was no one to take care of them, I would have to call DSS. She heard me say, "Call DSS," and she went ballistic. She came out of the room, hitting everybody, attacking the world—we had to call a Code 22 on her and had to wrestle her to the floor to give her medicine. I was the one rolling on the ground with her.

I talked to the police, and they told me the boyfriend was going to take care of the kids. When he came in, I said to him, "You know, we have to be sure that these kids are safe. Who's going to assume that responsibility?"

He said, "I take care of them a lot, so it's not a lot for me—the kids know me. I live there. I can take care of them."

I said, "We have to look for a long period of time—maybe two weeks. You need to go to work, and so, you need to think about how's this going to happen." He called the father of the children, and they made the arrangements to hand off the children. That worked out fine.

The patient ended up being admitted to a hospital, and she came back to see me about six weeks later. She was all cleaned up and doing well. She said, "I was so horrible to you," recalling the incident. She thanked me for treating her so respectfully. She was so grateful that it was enough to make you cry. She said the children were going to stay with their dad, and she was going to visit because she wasn't strong enough to take care of them yet. She just did a wonderful turnaround, and she was very grateful.

I actually called a physician at our associate hospital and told him the story. I remember that he did not seem to show the same degree of concern I did about this person. I believed she needed an emergent MRI. They weren't sure that she needed an emergent study right away because she looked fine; she was in no distress. He agreed to have the patient transferred.

I got feedback on her within an hour that her MRI showed a very large abscess that had continued to pinch on her spinal cord. It was actually the same physician who shook my hand the other day and said, "You know—you called it." So that was kind of nice.

I like to give some five-point details to the accepting physician on the other end. This is what I did, and this is what I think. It gives them a heads up as to how they might proceed. I remember calling the physician at the other hospital about the bleeding lady. I said, "Look, I really believe she has an intra-abdominal hemorrhage and she needs to be dealt with aggressively." I don't feel my responsibility ends as they go out the door. It's just like handing something off; you don't want the other person to be totally in the dark. So I want to at least give them my opinion as to what I feel needs to be done.

I guess the thing that delighted me most about the experience in the emergency room was the way it seemed like everyone there was focused on me. It was good because I felt awful, and everybody that came in was offering something. Do you want another pillow? Do you want this? Do you want that? They kept coming in to tell me what they were going to do. I didn't have to worry so I could sleep in between.

You always feel like you are the only one. You don't feel like a number here. You feel like they actually know you and that they really care.

When I first came into the emergency room, they didn't know what was wrong with me, and they refused to let me go home until they had some answers. Once they exhausted everything they could do, they asked to speak with my physician in Boston. They went through—I don't know how many numbers—until they finally reached her. They let my physician call the shots. They turned over all my medical care to her. She called in every hour, and they called her after every result came in. I thought that was absolutely amazing. My doctor completely ran the show, and they were more than happy to do that.

I guess the attention to my mom made me feel that they really cared. That was probably the most important thing, and I know it was to her too. She was exhausted from taking care of me and trying to convince my own doctors that I really was sick. That was probably the best.

I always knew what was going on. I was never sitting there wondering and waiting. I always knew how long the test should take and when the results would be in.

If they are busy, they'll say, "We haven't forgotten you. We are right here. We just had an emergency come in. Are you all set? Do you need anything right now? We won't be with you for awhile." They always keep you aware of what's going on. I found that very reassuring.

I get a different doctor every time I come to the ER, and each and every single one of them is wonderful.

The doctor told us where he went to school and a little bit about his background. It made us feel a little more comfortable. It made it easier for us to share personal details.

If you have a lab tech that needs to draw blood and you have X-rays that need to be done but you have to go to the bathroom, they listen to you. Both that nurse and that X-ray technician will wait for you. They will tell you, "'I'm here until 3:00 in the morning; take your time."

You are never waiting in a corridor cold and scared. You may wait in one room or the other, but you are never left out in a corridor. You are never completely alone either. There is always someone watching over you.

My mother was in the emergency room once from early morning until late at night. They treated her as nice at the end of the day as they did early in the morning.

Even though all of those rooms are filled, they come out and check you. They look at you and can tell if it's really a quick emergency. Last November I thought I was getting a urinary tract infection. You know how you can tell? You just have that feeling? Well, the ER was mobbed. I was dancing up and down. Someone asked me what was wrong. They just took care of me right away, even though they were so busy, because they knew I was so miserable.

Follow-Up Telephone Calls

My vision as manager was to enable the staff to see how their work made a difference. When I first introduced the idea of follow-up phone calls, the staff replied, "I can't believe you want us to do this now. What are you talking about?"

"I think it's a good thing," I told them. "It gives us a chance to see what's going on. Are the patients okay? Do they still have chest pain and need to come back?" We talked about it in the staff meetings, and then I approached many of them one on one. "Come on. We have to do it. Let's do it." Eventually they jumped on board.

We started simple. For example we'd call and say, "Jim, how are you doing? We just want to make sure you're doing okay." It is especially nice when they call the person they took care of because they know the whole story. Then I'm always happy when they get positive feedback. It makes the staff feel good, as well as the patients.

I had to police it at first. The first day, I said, "Did you do the follow-up calls?"

Staff replied, "No, I didn't have time."

"Well, let's try it after dinner," I suggested. I stayed there with them while they made a few calls. At times, I would go down to check on them, "Did you do follow-up calls?" If they said no I'd say, "Then you know what, you need to stop what you are doing and do the follow-up calls now, because it's not going away. I'll tell you what, I'll get somebody down to do the triage for you, so you can get the calls done." Eventually they realized it wasn't going away and they might as well get it done.

They continued to include the follow-up phone calls into their daily routine, and we were calling 90% of our patients back. It was going so well that the Joint Commission applauded our effort from a quality standpoint. They suggested we document the calls. Then the HIPAA rules came out, and I anticipated that there were going to be some problems with the new guidelines.

We now had to ask the patient when they came in if was okay to call them the next day. I had to come up with the whole thing of "how are we going to do this? What are we going to say? Where are we going to document on the chart that it's okay to call them?" To make all that work, I needed to give the staff extra encouragement to continue.

They said, "Let's skip the follow-up calls. It's just another thing we have to do, we're getting busier."

I told them we were not going to skip it. My role was to make the new process work and decide where on the chart it would be documented and to teach everybody how to do the asking.

Now we ask all of the patients if we can call them. As a result, we probably only call 50% now. Much of it has to do with the way the staff asks the question. I discovered that when nurses asked simply, "Can I call you tomorrow?" The patients asked, "Why?" They were reluctant to agree to the call. Many simply replied, "No." We found that if the staff posed the question differently, the patients usually agreed to the call. So, now our script is, "we usually try to call people the next day to see how they're doing. Is it okay to call you?" My vision is to try to get that back up to 90%.

There was a day not too long ago that the nurse was doing follow-up calls and was busy and really didn't want to do them—just way too busy. I got some help from another unit to take care of patients while she did the calls. One of the patients she called said, "That little sweetheart that took care of me, she was so nice. I don't know her name, but you make sure that she . . . (it was the nurse making the call!). You make sure that that young lady gets a big thank you from me because she was just the nicest person. You know, she helped me to the car."

When I heard about this, I said to that nurse, "See? And you didn't want to call her."

The nurse said, "I know."

The staff reports that it is a little bit time consuming, but assuming I was the patient on the other end of the phone, I would be happy to hear from the nurse who saw me. Also, we realize that it is a big, big plus for this place. Now that we have to ask if we can call, I hear people say, "I can't believe you guys do this; it is so fantastic!"

Each call is a little different. It depends on how much reinforcement you need to do. A lot of times when patients are here, they don't always hear everything at discharge. The phone calls follow through with that. Some patients say they are fine and "goodbye." Others want to chat and you have to say, "Glad you're doing well, have a good day."

We find the time in between patients as much as we can. Sometimes you pick up that stack of patients that need to be called, and you can't do it. It stays there because the patient coming in is your priority. We rely on our supervisor to have staff from other units to help us. We pass the stack on from one shift to another if we can't finish them. Everyone tries to finish them.

I seem to do a lot of them some days, and I've had a lot of patients who will thank me right away. "Oh, thank you so much for calling. That was so nice of you." They get that sense that we care beyond their visit here. It's not that we sent them home and that's the end of it. We ask, "How are you doing today? Did you get through the night? Do you have any questions? Make sure you follow-up with your doctor." It just goes beyond what we do here—we extend to them.

Family

A strength our staff has is their approach to patient care. There is a culture here of caring about people like they are family. They remember the patient. It's Mrs. Jones, or Bertha, or Rita, or Jack, or whatever, and not "the one down in 22" or "the one over here" or "the gallbladder." They remember people and treat people like they're family.

I try to treat every child like they are my own. It makes them feel like they are taken care of.

I think most of us come in here with the attitude that anybody we see could be your mother, your father, or a very dear friend. So, you take care of them as if they were. If you focus on patients that way, you will do your best.

I always try to think that this could be my mother or father or grandmother in the bed and treat them how I would want my family to be treated.

I like the fact that you can go to lunch and sit at the same table with the senior leadership, and you can just have a casual conversation. There's no stress—nothing. I like that. I also like that we have The Fling; everyone's birthdays are listed there, and we can say happy birthday to everyone.

What I like about it most is it's a very friendly atmosphere no matter where you go. It is almost like working with family.

I remember when we were almost closed down because we were going to go bankrupt. The worst part wasn't that people lost their jobs; they kind of lost their family, too.

They really care about what they're doing. We can disagree on many things, but at the end of the day, we all agree on what we're here for. They do it, not only with patients, but they do it with their coworkers. I often tell people it's like a family: They can rip you to shreds one minute and bicker the way families always do, but should you have a problem or an issue, they will just rally right around and make sure they take care of you. So, they care about their patients; they care about each other.

I think Clinton's core value that needs to be preserved is its strong sense of community. When I think about that I think about that song from *Cheers* where everybody knows your name. That makes me think of Clinton Hospital.

Employee Selection

The essence of Clinton Hospital is clearly the people. We need to make sure we are looking for people who share our values and make an effort to keep them here and promote them through. I think that's a piece of it.

We have a low turnover rate, a low callout rate, and people who are willing to pick up extra shifts. Of people who work in the ER, very few leave. They stay. That says something to me. I think that's success.

When you apply for a job here, you get a prompt response. Within hours, that application is in the appropriate person's mailbox. We in HR make sure we get the people connected with the managers as soon as possible. Sometimes the manager will come down the same day that the person walks in. They talk to them about the position, availability, and expectations. One new employee reports, "I knew right away that these people really were interested in me. They thought I was kind of important the day I walk in the door."

I went online just looking for jobs and saw that they had a 32-hour position open here. I said, "Oh, what the heck. I'll e-mail my resume." So I e-mailed my resume, and within two hours they called me for an interview!

One of the managers who works here is a manager that I recruited. She was a nurse I went to nursing school with, and I thought she would do a wonderful job. I was thinking it would be nice to have someone here that has the same work ethic as me. There was an opening on the second floor. She said she was interested. I spoke to the VP of nursing at the time. I remember I wanted to sell her because I felt like she would do a really good job. I felt like she had the "meat and potatoes" of what we were looking for.

The VP's response, which I didn't expect, was, "You know, it's not good to work with friends. If you disagree, then that spills over into your outside relationship."

I said that I thought we could handle that. I remember leaving the meeting thinking that when she meets my friend, she's going to like her. I trusted she would sell herself.

Indeed, she came to work here, does a magnificent job, and is a great support. If I need help, she will take care of everything. I think that's key. You have to have someone there if you need it.

I fell down a flight of stairs a week ago, Saturday. I mean I went down the whole flight of stairs. Messed up my leg—came in hobbling. Not only did she try to do all of the running for me, but also, she said, "You need to go home and I'll take care of this."

I said, "Okay." She just took care of everything. She knows the place well, so, I don't have to tell her.

Orientation Welcome

A new employee is a valuable asset, and it is our obligation to make that employee feel welcome and give them the tools that they need to do their job. We need to get them settled and integrated into a department. We value them as an important member of our team. We want to keep them here. We want to do everything to have them be happy here.

Although it's not necessarily our jobs in human resources, we support department managers in that role. We visit the employees, acknowledge them, meet them, talk with them, and ask them how they are doing. We check with the managers to see how they are doing. "Is there anything we can do to help this particular candidate?" This is especially true in the ER, which can be a very challenging area to staff. We even celebrate when the ER manger has her full staff.

We just had a luncheon for some new hires. We do it on a quarterly basis. We bring in new employees at about the three-month mark, along with people who have been here for about a year, just to talk about how things are going. "Are you getting what you need? Are things working in the department?" We let them know, "We are happy to have you here. We would like to hear about any issues." Also, please tell us the good things you have experienced so that we can share them with the department.

We hear stories from new employees that they came in and felt welcomed into the environment. They feel comfortable and supported. For example, a gentleman said today that he could "ask anybody anything about the process here and all were more than willing to help. People understood that I was new and needed some assistance."

As the physician director, my bottom line feeling about physicians who come out to this ED to work is that they should not do things to move us backward. Their personalities should be such that they are going to help us move forward. They cannot undo what it has taken years to do. I say to new employees, "Just remember this is a community hospital. We are very much part of this community. What you say matters to these patients, and how you say it matters to the patients."

The family setting is very important to new employees. One new employee did use the term *family*, and I think that really says she walked in and felt welcomed. That people took her under their wing—helped her learn things.

They've made me feel welcome. They will do anything for you, switching time and all that kind of stuff.

I came here about 11 years ago, and I really only planned to stay about a year. Here I am 11 or 12 years later. I was really impressed with the people that I worked with and how everyone really works as a team. I found that the hospital had a real heart and soul and really cared about its patients and employees.

You know how you are on eggshells for a while because you are still new? You are not quite sure you are doing things right. When I was new someone said to me, "You are doing a really good job, and we can see that you are growing and you are getting more confidence." I was thrilled. I went home and told my husband, "They like me honey, they like me." I was on cloud nine.

Leadership Sets the Tone

One of the things is that you sort of set a tone. The team follows the tone of the leader. I think that is true almost in any species.

I think you need to have managers who are out of the pumps and pearls and who manage at the bedside and see what's going on. You can't be the coach of the football team if you've never been on the team, nor can you coach the team from your kitchen. You need to see what's going on. You need to see how they're reacting with the patients so that if it's not good you can correct it. If you're in your kitchen, you can't see how that happens.

We need to have managers who can be there and feel it and know it. I think we always try to, and one of the things administration does do here is listen to the staff. I think you have to be down there to hear the staff. If you get too big and too fluffy, you miss it. You're not going to hear it.

The CEO happened by the ER when they were particularly busy. A staff member called out, "I didn't get lunch. Can you get me a sandwich?"

She said, "Sure. No problem."

I think that what's important for this team is that we routinely sit down and talk with each other. We try to meet on a regular basis. I think the way you structure the environment helps. If you have people right next door to each other, generally they are going to talk to each other more.

I support the managers and the staff by providing them what they need. It is my job. If I don't hear them, I can't get them the resources they need. If I'm not working on their behalf, if I'm not helping them be successful in their job, then I am not doing mine.

We had a three month old come in that we worked on and really worked hard with. I was thinking that this wasn't going to be a good outcome. If you've got a baby who's not breathing and has no pulse on the outside, he or she is not coming back.

The doctor wanted to call it and I told him, "You can't call it yet until that mother comes here. She needs to see us actively working on her baby before we call it." He was okay with that suggestion because he knew it was the right thing.

When the mother came in, I told the mother what had happened. "The baby sitter found the baby not breathing and called 911. The baby is still not breathing despite all that we did, and even if we breathe for the baby, his little heart isn't beating. We have given him medicine, and it's not looking like his heart is going to start." So, she has time to think about this a little bit. We're still doing CPR, and we gave the baby some more medicine. So, she had 10 minutes to be there.

My role is to make sure everybody is doing his or her job. You can't have somebody there who gets so caught up in the emotion of the moment that they stand there crying. You need to get out of there. On that day, we had a couple of nurses with tears in their eyes. I said, "You know what? No time for that. You need to. . . ." Like cold-hearted Anna, "You need to regroup. If you can't stay here, then you leave, and we'll get a substitute. Right now. That's it. Get a grip on it."

At the debriefing, we had all of the nurses and respiratory therapists and lab—all of the people that were involved. The doctor that was involved in that care [was there], and the social worker actually ran it. At the debriefing, one of the greatest things that I had was the respiratory therapist who had worked in a large teaching facility and she had been involved in other SIDS deaths. She had never seen such care given to the family and the baby as was given in our ER. That did it for me. That was good.

The new equipment we had just purchased wasn't compatible with the old equipment. In a stressful situation like this one, you don't want to yell, "Oh, we've got the wrong blades!" That will turn the stress up for everybody else.

We quickly found the equipment that worked. Afterward, we knew we had to fix the problem. We told the leadership about the situation, and they said, "It won't happen again. We will order new equipment." It wasn't a question of how much was it going to cost. We were on the same page.

My feeling is really not a matter of "should have knowns." You never want a problem to end as "they should have known." You want to look at a situation and ask, "How can we make it as easy as possible to know?" It's just like an extremely well-trained pilot going through a checklist. It would be inappropriate to say they know the things by heart, and thus, they shouldn't have to go down the checklist. Going through the process eliminates errors.

One thing that stands out about communication is rounding. Our 3–11 staff sometimes leaves at midnight. We had a designated parking area for them where they felt comfortable going out when they get off shift. We found our day shift staff was parking there. This sounds like a simple problem. You will just tell people to not park there. That didn't work.

So, through rounding on the shifts and meeting with some of the different staff, we talked about caring about each other. Instead of just saying "that is 3–11 parking," I try talking to them about how some of the evening staff might feel.

We need to think about how *they* feel about it. They are your co-workers. Quite frankly, the 3–11 staff is coming in and relieving you guys on days, so, you want them to come in happy. We probably want to think about why we take their parking place. They are going to be upset when they come in. What we are saying to them is this: "We don't care about you so we park in your parking place."

We had to have that discussion at more than one staff meeting, a couple of months apart. The last time I rounded I actually was able to go to the different meetings and say, "You know what? You're showing you care." The day staff isn't parking there any more.

I met with all of the staff of one department and asked about issues. They said there was not enough staff. They didn't feel like they could take vacation. It was just not worth it. I thought, "They shouldn't feel that way. We need to fix this problem." We did. We gave them another full-time position.

I think the important thing is that we responded to what they were telling us and that the manager was able to feel like he advocated for his staff—that he listened and that administration listened. They were thrilled with the response.

There was an older lady who was not a frequent visitor but had sought medical help for back pain three times recently. I needed to look at this lady more closely. The lady was very friendly, not in any type of distress. I wasn't sure she had a critical issue, but my threshold of concern was high because she had a low-grade temperature. I guess I have enough experience not to get too concerned about what other people think might be my clinical threshold or my concern.

We recently, in the past year, worked very hard on getting a new CAT scan machine in here. It is a million-dollar project, which is huge for a small hospital. If we were going to be vital to the community, if we were going to grow, we had to find a way to fund this project.

So my job was to coax the CFO to really sit down and do an analysis of how we could fund this thing, where we could take money from, and how we could potentially do it. There was a lot of coaxing and that sort of thing. I knew he was going to do it eventually. You obviously have to change the way you work with people, depending on what you're dealing with.

We completed it this year, and I think it is probably one of the greatest things that we have done for Clinton in terms of preparing it for the future.

There is open communication between management and all of us in every department. We have monthly meetings with our CEO, and she wants to hear about anything—if there are ants in the vending machine room to the parking issues. So, open communication is great.

Coaching and Being Coached

I first got involved with coaching one of our administrative people five or six years ago. I was thinking she was going to be a wonderful nurse. She decided to leave to attend nursing school. When she came back, she worked in the ICU but was very shaky. She grew a little bit there and then transferred to the ED. The first couple of years she was good, but not really solid. We worked together, and I would tell her things she needed to do differently.

When I saw situations where she seemed intimidated, I would ask, "Why did you feel uncomfortable doing that?" For example, after a code situation, I would say, "Why didn't you start that IV? You know you can do it. You need to feel more confident." She was really insecure. I continued to encourage her with comments like, "You can do this. You know you can do this. You *need* to be able to do this. Think about this now, work on it." I always told her she could do it—never told her she couldn't.

She began to show more confidence. I was thinking, "This kid's got it. She just needs to get her feet on the ground, and I'm going to help her do that." I felt as though she had the ability to be a really good nurse. I thought, "She's great; she's one of my best nurses. I just needed to help her get her feet on the ground." Now she can run the whole show down there. She can be the person in charge and has taken on other duties.

We have a very kind, hard-working physician who is concerned about his patients, but was getting negative feedback from patients. He is a very quiet person, and I think that that mislead people to believe that he was not listening. So we set into motion a process. I sat him down, and I said, "We need to fix this." We needed to make this right because it is real important to patients. I suggested some steps he should take. First, I told him, pull up a chair by the patient before you start asking questions. That immediately sends the message, "I'm listening. I'm going to spend a minute extra here." Second, introduce yourself to the family members as well as the patient. Tell them you are concerned not only about the patient, but also what they think. Third, repeat what you say, and ask them if they understand what you are saying. As a result, he improved a great deal, and we have seen a real reduction in the number of complaint letters.

As EMTs on ambulance calls, we get to talk to the doctor after he sees the patient. You can go over and ask him questions about what's going on, and he'll sit there and talk to you for 5–10 minutes so that you know what's going on with the patient. If you have any questions, you can ask anything that we could have done differently during the process.

They provide us with the opportunity to observe, to learn, to ask questions, and to feel comfortable doing it. You don't feel like if you say something or speak up that you are going to get your head chopped off or somebody is going to be better than you are. It's just a good rapport. They treat us with respect.

When I first started as an EMT student, I came to Clinton Hospital to observe. The respiratory therapist basically took me under his wing and brought me around and showed me how to use his equipment. He encouraged me to help him with patients but also encouraged me to work on patient interaction. It was a very good place for me to learn, developing that rapport with patients. He basically just took me under his wing the entire time I was here, and you don't get that one-on-one attention anywhere else.

An important relationship I've built here at Clinton Hospital is with my nurse manager. She really mentored me to this new role. Even though she had so much more experience than I, she showed a great deal of deference to my role as medical director. I had never been involved in anything administrative before, and I really looked at how she dealt with problems, how she dealt with her nurses, and the standard that she expected not only from herself but also from all her nurses. This was an uncompromising standard that took into account the individual limitations of people's own personal lives and their own personal limitations. She demanded the best that each person could be, within their capacity. This was a hugely important thing for me to see.

She also has a great way of saying, "You know, I really think we should try this. I really think you should look at this. What do you think of this? What is your opinion?" It really allowed me to grow rather than be overrun by somebody who had a lot more experience.

When I conduct performance appraisals, I ask my staff to give me feedback, either in writing or verbally. "I've shared with you my impressions about how I think you are doing. Now I want you tell me how you think *I'm* doing."

This doctor came in, nice looking, very pleasant, but he stood in the room and he said to me, "Well, I just want you to know up front that I don't really treat geriatrics. So you are going to need to. . . ." One of the nurses interrupted him and said, "Can I see you for a minute?" She took him right outside. "Don't you ever talk to a patient like that! Whether you treat them or not, when you are in front of that patient, you better be. . . ." Here was this little tiny nurse telling this guy. I thanked her for that because my mom did hear it.

We had a difficult call several months ago, the chief of police and the husband of the patient called life flight without going through the usual channels. There was another critically ill patient in the emergency room at the time that the staff had already called life flight for. There was some disagreement about which patient would need the air transport. As EMTs, we were caught in the middle. The ED doctor later took us aside and took the time to explain to us that the whole situation was handled poorly. We really appreciated that he told us how we could have handled it a little differently. He understood the circumstances of the pressure that we were under.

Teamwork

I feel that everybody rolls up their sleeves and pitches in when the going gets tough. Often times they step out of their job to help. If there is housekeeping that needs to be done and there is no housekeeper, there is not an employee here who wouldn't mop a floor. It is not uncommon for a nurse's aid from another unit to stop by the ED and make up a stretcher on her way to get coffee.

Any area knows they may have to help another area immediately. People can flex very quickly, with many people coming into a situation. People know when they need to be somewhere. Nurses will just migrate somewhere and know that they have to stay. These steps and processes are just honed from years of doing them, and a lot of credit goes to the nurse manager for developing that sense of responsibility among her nurses. The way they can handle a couple of things simultaneously and understand how to shift.

We wanted to re-look at the structure of the ED. It was designed in a different time when different rules and different paradigms applied. One of the small rooms we have was designated as a procedure room. We noticed, "You know, we have two people who have cuts. We can only manage one, and one is sitting out in the waiting room. Why don't we try to move our rooms around? Let's rethink what we do here. Why don't we try to restructure our rooms so that we can make a larger room our procedure room? That way we can have two beds." So, just between our conversations we agreed.

Our collaborative relationship focused on our shared vision for the ER. We didn't want it to be just what it was; we wanted it to grow into the best that we could make it. We looked at it not only from the standpoint from patient care and medical care, but also the secretarial staff, the patient comfort level, and the waiting room level.

If I'm not busy with patients, I'm stocking. I'm organizing, or I'm cleaning. I know that the people on the next shift appreciate it because there have been comments made like, "Boy what a difference when she's on. When we get here we aren't stocking all night. Most of it's done."

They need to be here. They need to participate, and they need to be team players. If you can't be a team player, you can't participate. Bottom line—you need to part of the whole. You need to be part of how we supply the place, how we clean the place. You need to be on that team, and we make that very clear.

The staff in my units work together to fix their schedule around special occasions. Once I post the time, they swap with each other. So, I don't have to get into that whole mess of "she's always looking for time." They work that out together so that one pays the other and its reciprocal. They all sort of get the feel that they belong to this department. They own it.

I called up one of the nurses; she came in, lives local. She was here in 15 minutes, and she essentially stayed with that patient until she was discharged. So, she stayed more than two hours. She probably stayed four or five hours.

In the lab, we work kind of behind the scenes most of the time. We don't really see any patients, and we rely totally on you guys. The feedback that we get from all of you, from the front lines, is good. That's why we stay here. You know who we are even though you never see us, but it is the way everybody works together that's what keeps us going. You are our world, and you're great!

I think that there is a certain level of comfort with someone that you can just sort of sit down and be yourself with. You don't have to think that you have to say the right thing or you have to do the right thing. You don't feel that that person is going to be criticizing you the minute you walk out the door. There is a certain level of trust.

I have a colleague who always provides all of the details we need on a project. She is more detail oriented than I am, much more detail oriented. I have seen her notes before; I have seen her talk with people before. She is very thorough, and I know I can trust her to deliver.

We really do support one another. This patient came in one night, really sick, vomiting. That night, we had the doctor, the nurse, the supervisor, the lab tech, the housekeeper, life flight, and a toxicologist working on this patient. The next day, the day shift said, "Don't worry about the cleanup. Don't worry about stocking. You go home. We'll take care of that." I always value that teamwork.

Rewards and Recognition

I think the hospital must own a movie theater or something because we have been thanked with movie tickets. I don't know why, but it is very nice. There seems to be a trend here.

I've had a couple of my ER nurses come in and worked up in the unit when they really didn't want to. It's not their area of expertise, you know. I've had a couple that have come in and worked an extra Saturday and stayed late and whatever. So you know what I do? I give them movie tickets. I give them tickets to the movies, and I give them a little letter; the little letter that says, "Thank you so much for going above and beyond the call of duty. When you came in last Friday, I don't know what I would have done without your help. I know this isn't a lot, but I just want to say that I really appreciate the fact of what you do." I cc it to their personnel file, and I send them two tickets to the movies or send them those gift coupons for Dunkin' Donuts.

Part of the community feeling here is when we've had good inspections. The "big guns" aren't afraid to say, "Congratulations! Let's go out and celebrate." The president of the hospital and the administration staff took us out. That's part of the family thing. It is just fabulous. I appreciate that a lot.

We recently had a joint commission lab survey, and we celebrated actually with the whole staff. We got to celebrate a little bit with them, to tell them how proud we were of the work that they did. They want the leadership to be there and celebrate with them. I think that's important. I think it is important that we can adapt to two kinds of celebrations—the one that they really enjoy, the more informal one, and then do it in a formal way here. I think that says something to that whole group.

We did an ice cream sundae in the cafeteria for the staff, and everybody in the hospital was invited to go down and have some ice cream and talk about the great job that everybody did. People loved it. It's our favorite. It's certainly a small token of our appreciation. It has been an effective way that we've found to recognize people for various types of occasions.

We actually had an employee meeting, and we reviewed some of the results of the Press Ganey scores, both outpatient and emergency departments. We had a cake; we gave everybody some cake and congratulated them all. We told them how they all made this work for the hospital and where we wanted to go next. We did that on all three shifts, brought the cake around, and told everybody the results and how they all contributed to those results.

Every time I get a thank you note from a patient—we get a lot of those—I look it up, and I see who the nurse and doctor were who took care of them. I write their names on the card so that they get the kudos. You like to get those.

My boss will write a little note of thanks, and she'll tell me what a wonderful job I do. But that's not why I do it. I do it to hopefully make a difference to someone.

Extending to Community

We communicate regularly with the primary care doctors. We give them information about their patients in real time as much as possible, and they give it back to us. It's the same thing with the patients.

The fire department was invited to the debriefing after an infant died. They had to hold a dead baby and do CPR on a dead baby. The fireman that participated never had to do that before, so that was very painful for him. He told me afterward that it was good for him to talk about it. I knew he needed to talk about it. I've seen this a few times and know that they need to talk about it because, you know, babies don't die every day. It's not something that happens every day of the week. That's why it is good for them to have to talk about it.

Our ambulance crews have done two disaster drills with the ED, and afterward, they invited us up here and actually took our input and let us critique how their emergency department worked. We suggested other ways we can make it run smoother in a drill like that in a disaster. You will see things change based on our suggestions.

The various departments, along with the ER staff, are all one great big happy family. When we come in with someone critical, if they are short handed, they always let you go right in the room with them, to bag or whatever, until their staff gets up to speed. It just gives you a rewarding feeling that you are part of the team.

They go out to the ambulance and meet us. I've worked several codes where I've never had to lift anyone out of the ambulance because they are pulling them right out, and you are still a part of it. I actually had a nurse say, "Don't leave me." I was fine with that. It makes you feel appreciated. You know that they understand your job and appreciate it.

When we've taken the time to get patients in a collar, they don't pull it off as soon as we get there. They respect what we've done. They don't question us. They wait until the X-rays are done to remove the collar.

I think a big part of it is they don't mind us being there, observing. We come in. We are always asking questions and they are always willing to give us an answer. They explain what they are doing and why they are doing it.

One of the things that I like about working with the staff here is that if we ask them what contributed to the incident, they are willing to tell us what happened. They tell us what they did and what the outcome was and whether they were transferred to another hospital. Those are the things that we like to know and find out.

Last week we lost a member of our department—our EMS coordinator. It was very gratifying to see all of these people from the surrounding towns and a lot of the doctors and nurses at the funeral. The church was full. I was amazed. I was thinking to myself, "Who's left at the hospital?"

Even a busy surgeon will stop and show and explain to us just what is going on. We recently had a construction worker who put a nail gun through his knee. We brought him in and did the paperwork. Shortly after that, we were able to go in and see the X-ray, and the surgeon showed us the impact of where the nail had gone and what they were going to do.

The medical director also helps us in other ways. Every year he does a drill, a training session, at our Christmas party. We have fun and get credit at the same time. He takes the time to come out and to do this. He doesn't get paid for it; he does this all on his own. So, it's "dine and defib" tonight (laughter). Ho! Ho! Ho!

We are all just an extension of the hospital.

Above and Beyond

People step outside their typical role to help out. We don't deliver babies here, but about twice a year someone surprises us. Maybe a year and half after I started here, a woman came in ready to deliver. She was having her baby in the emergency department. One of the things that impressed me were two internists who left their offices and came down to help this woman. We called them, and they came in a minute. It was not something they *had* to do; as a matter of fact, they may have even taken some risk coming, given that they are not OB/GYN doctors. The staff dealt wonderfully with the mother and baby, and all were happy with the care. It's a great story and is the typical job the staff would do.

One of the case managers has worked with patients here for many years, generally works with inpatients or ED patients who need placement. I've actually seen her sitting in the lobby counseling and helping people from the community who are not patients in the hospital.

She frequently gets requests like, "Can you come to the lobby? Mr. so-and-so is here and would like to speak with you." This isn't part of her day-to-day job, and although it does take up some of her time, she will spend the time to get them information they need. I've not only seen her do that with people in the community, but for employees also. I think that's important and I think this kind of thing happens throughout the organization, not just in her case.

One patient tells of the time she came to the ED with her boyfriend. "We dislocated a shoulder again," she announced. As the physician was trying to manipulate the shoulder, she said to him, "Last time we came in the doctor had him lay on his chest, hang his arms and put a weight around it. That really worked, if you want to try it." The doctor agreed. So I'm running around the ER getting the weights and putting them on. He had no problem with me showing him what worked before. He even said, "Boy that did work. I've never seen that before." It amazed me that a doctor let someone like me show him how to do his job. He was willing to do whatever it took to make it work.

They just stick their neck out for you. This patient had arrived at the ED by ambulance in severe pain from a beating. In the confusion, a police officer had mistakenly assumed that this patient had tried to harm her children. There was another nurse taking care of somebody else two gurneys away who heard all the commotion and knew that the officer was under the wrong impression. The patient remembers that "the nurse came flying around and she stuck her nose into a place where she probably shouldn't have, but she knew that my kids should not be allowed to go with their father. I have no idea who she was."

Her friend later said to her, "There was an angel looking out for you tonight. . . . There was a nurse who stuck her nose in because of what she overheard." The patient said, "If she hadn't stuck her nose in, I was told that he would have resumed custody, and I would have had to go to court to fight to get them back."

I work at a funeral home, and oftentimes we will have the nurses here who will come in because they've had the patient in the ER or up on the floor and they will actually come into the wake. You should see the family's faces when they see their nurses! They will come through with their uniforms or scrubs on and that family feels absolutely marvelous when they see them come in. It happened this morning. One of the nurses came in.

Yeah, my staff, they're pretty good. I can just call them up and say, "You know what, gang? We're all sort of jammed up here for a little while. Can you give me a couple of hours?"

I said "Here's the story—we need a little help now. Can you help me for a couple of hours and I'll try to get you out of this as soon as possible." And they come in.

I've even had two nurses who gave up part of their vacation on Cape Cod to come and work. In fact, they offered. When they saw that I would be in trouble with staffing during their vacation, they offered to each come back and cover some of the shifts.

Actually, those two who gave up vacation came in and said, "Whoa. You have no staffing. Even if you work every day, you're still going to be in trouble."

I said, "No kidding. Everything that could go wrong did go wrong."

They said, "What are you going to do?"

I said, "Well, any and all help is greatly appreciated. Got any ideas?"

They said they would work. So, they both worked. I got a letter off to them. I was going to get them a case of beer, but I thought that was not going to cut it. I sent them to Dunkin' Donuts. I gave them things for Dunkin' Donuts because they're both big Dunkin' Donuts fans. Even little things like that. Now, both of those people work at another facility, and they saved the letters and gave them to the boss over there, and said, "This is what happens at a real hospital." Both of those were big hospitals—really big teaching hospitals.

It was a weekend night—I want to say maybe a Sunday night—and we had this gentleman come in with chest pain. He needed a chest tube before we transported him. It was right at the change of shift. I offered to stay on later than my shift. Thankfully, the supervisor told me that I could stay, and the overtime was approved. I wanted this patient to have the same nurse follow the whole thing through until transport. I think that makes a big difference to the patient. The family knew that my shift ended at 11, so when it got close to midnight they said, "What are you still doing here? You were supposed to leave!" I told them I was not going to leave them in midstream. They were so thankful. The wife gave me a hug. It made me feel good that they appreciated my staying.

Warm Blanket

Everybody knows about the warm blanket. The difference here is you have time to give that warm blanket. About 10 years ago, the ER manager commandeered the blanket warmer from the OR when they purchased a new one. It is a commonly heard term throughout the organization—both literally and figuratively.

My friend couldn't be at this focus group tonight because she is in the hospital! She called me from her bedside to say, "Please tell them my story!" Yesterday, as soon as we walked in to the ER, she was cold. She said, "I'm cold." It's frightening to come to an emergency room because you don't know what is going to happen. They put that warm Johnny on her, and that little smile came to her face. She felt so much better.

I bring a patient back from radiology to the ER and I'm like, "Are you cold? Do you want a blanket?" I give them a warm blanket. I treat them just as nice as anything.

I remember lying on the bed in the middle of the night feeling really sick. This janitor or something went and got my mom a blanket, one of the warm blankets. That was really nice.

The patient was shivering, so they gave her a warm blanket. "Take it out of the oven and wrap her up."

Yeah. It makes them feel good. It makes them feel like someone's caring and thinking about them. It's just a little extra step.

That's a great machine they got down there. We are always using it—just grab a blanket. We (the EMTs) are allowed to use the warm blankets. We had a patient the other night. It was raining. He was soaked and wet, and he was shivering. They said, "Okay, get the blankets." We put the blankets on him and he felt much better then.

The first thing we did was get him a couple blankets out of the warmer, and it was great. That's what he needed.

Then they put a warm blanket on you also, and then if you say, "I'm cool or cold," they put another warm blanket on you. I thought that was great.

I remember one experience about a warm blanket at a time when we were really, really busy. I noticed that a lady was chilled when I was walking by. I asked her if she wanted a warm blanket, and she said, "Yes, can I please get one?" I gave it to her, walked away, and didn't think anything of it. Later on, I was at a church service being introduced to a lady who said, "Oh, yeah, I know her. She's the girl at the hospital that gave me the warm blanket. You don't know how much you helped me out that day. It was just nice. Everyone was running around. They were busy, and you thought to give me the warm blanket."

We need to preserve that wonderful blanket warmer that we have in the ER, and it's the nicest thing for these old folks or anyone who has been in a car accident that we have this nice warm blanket that we wrap around them.

We want to preserve in essence the warm blanket—the good feeling that patient's get when they're here.

Editor Commentary

Working as a team is necessary for the delivery of great emergency care, and the physicians, nurses, clinicians, support staff, and EMTs associated with Clinton Hospital offer multiple examples of how to generate the trust and camaraderie necessary for a team to function at the highest levels. Staff members cited numerous examples of feeling valued for their unique perspectives, talents, and contributions—no matter what their formal roles. They exhibit a high level of trust in each other and confidence in each other's abilities.

The feeling of collegiality and ease of working together appears to be fostered by a particularly adept ED manager. Emergency care is stressful work, perhaps the most stressful environment in all of health care. The hands-on leadership and role modeling demonstrated by the unit leader and her attention to helping the staff keep a good balance between their work lives and personal lives have a positive impact on the team members. The ED manager takes a personal interest in the lives of the members and accommodates their unique needs, and as a result, the staff members feel valued and respected. This, in turn, generates their loyalty to the department, to the organization, and to each other. The care they all take with orientation and helping a new team member feel welcomed and supported seems critical to their success as well.

The vision and directive of the senior leadership team to "put patients first" is manifested in numerous stories and examples from the team of "going above and beyond" to serve patients, families, and visitors. They related an obvious pleasure in their ability to make a difference and share a resounding pride in their own efforts and those of their colleagues as well. Patients reported feeling the difference, mentioning numerous times that they felt the staff really cared about them as unique individuals, not as "a number." Clearly, the warm blankets work—for the staff, the EMTs, and the patients, too. Staff members felt supported by the leadership—being empowered to act and having the resources made available to them. They are interested in and committed to asking questions about how can we learn more and get better. The leaders at all levels have high expectations; they celebrate and acknowledge the group's successes and simultaneously challenge the team to continuously improve their processes.

The story of implementing follow-up phone calls seems to be a good indicator of their successful approach to improvement. The leader chose this activity to connect with the staff and their ability to make a difference and receive the positive comments about their skills and ability. With any change in habits, however, it takes more than issuing a memo. The leader's continued coaching, focus on the positive results, unshakable setting of expectations, and engagement of the staff in making improvements in the process have resulted in an artifact that would be the envy of most emergency departments.

Table 6-1 Organizational Demographics

Organization	Cleveland Clinic, Fairview Hospital
Location	Cleveland, OH
Setting	Suburban
Communities served	Suburban and urban
Type of organization	Nonprofit community hospital, teaching hospital (nursing and medical residents)
Number of Beds	486
Number of FTEs	2,849
Scope of service	ER Trauma Level II, Neonatal Intensive Care, Women's and Obstetrics Level III (highest), Gastrointestinal Disorders, Invasive Cardiology, Oncology, Skilled Nursing, Cardiac Rehab, Pediatrics, Pediatrics ER, Inpatient and Outpatient Medical Surgical, Intensive Care, Coronary Care, Respiratory Care, Radiology, Family Practice, Orthopedics, Pathology, Anesthesia, Occupational Therapy/Physical Therapy
Organizational awards	Solucient Award (Nation's Top 100 Hospitals)
	North Coast 99 Award (Best Place to Work in 2005 and 2006)
	Ernest Codman Award (effective use of performance measures) (2001 and 2003)
	NRC Survey—consistently in the top 10% nationwide
Focus area	Environmental Services Department
Focus area	Environmental Services received the Cleveland Clinic "World Class Service Teamwork Award"
Best practices and awards	NRC—top 10% nationwide for the last 5 years Employee satisfaction in the top 5% nationally for the past 5 years
	Cleveland Clinic patient callback program has been the leader since its inception

CHAPTER 6

The Listening Business

Contributor: Robert E. Cannon

The stories in this chapter are the voices of senior leadership at the Cleveland Clinic, Fairview Hospital senior leadership, director and assistant director of Environmental Services, housekeeping staff, and patients. Here are their stories.

FAIRVIEW HOSPITAL: A CLEVELAND CLINIC HOSPITAL

People First

I care about the people I work with. The work we do is very important, but the creation of relationships at all levels is what I value most.

My office is a barrier. My title is a barrier, and even the way you get to my office is a barrier. Despite all of the barriers, a year ago the leader of the Cardiac Cath Lab came to my office to tell me about one of her staff members who was a unit secretary and whose mother was dying in Hungary. She just didn't have the resources to be with her mother, and the staff was concerned that this moment in her life was really important to her. What could we do to help? I thought about it a little, and I said, "We have resources." The staff at each of our hospitals had created the Employee Care Fund for employees in their time of need. So, with the help of the chief administrative officer of the hospital, we put together a program that utilized some organizational resources and money from the Employee Care Fund. We will hold this person harmless while they are away so that it will not negatively impact the family. We can make those decisions here, and that is kind of nice.

It was an important event because our organization only works at its optimum when our staff members understand that its first customer is each other. To reach out to each other is extraordinarily important and creates a great organization. It shows that the patient in lots of ways isn't first. The doctor isn't first, and even the community isn't first. It is creating a community of supporting caregivers that makes a great hospital and a great organization. We were able to financially help this person. A lot of wonderful things have happened, but that was clearly the top.

Fairview is different. Fairview is unique. Administration believes in doing the right thing, and they care very much about the employees. If you talk to our CEO very long, you will notice that probably 80% of his conversations are about one thing. You take care of the employees. You treat them with respect, and you value them. Those are my values as well. I have a passion for people. I feel comfortable here. I feel valued and appreciated. That is important.

Something I learned as a director is that I can't move the patient satisfaction scores until I move the employee satisfaction scores first. Once we meet their needs, then they are able to meet the needs of our patients.

Common thinking is that patients come first, and that is the ultimate thing to do. Our CEO says that in order to be able to put patients first, you need to make sure that everybody else is okay. So he talks about taking care of each other. It doesn't necessarily mean me taking care of staff that reports to me— it means the guy next to you, too. We are not there yet, but that is a great goal—to have everybody watching everybody else's back. If your immediate needs are taken care of, only then can you take care of somebody else's needs.

Believing in People

It is really important for leaders to direct the spotlight at the right things. By doing that you say to everybody, in a really effective way, what is valued. If you are leading the right way (the effective way), people know it. If I don't value good performance, what does that tell everyone else? Telling stories is motivating. It is fulfilling to be around people doing good things.

We find examples of great care—great support of each other and republish them. Instead of saying we need to be the best place to work, I write stories about what is the best place to work. Instead of saying we do great patient care, I will share letters from patients. I write something once a week for our staff.

We have an extremely competent and bright group of people. They really have a great sense of why we are here. I enjoy working with them because they get it. I think we have the right people.

I try to help everyone be all that they can be through a systematic approach. While I hold them accountable, I also help them to improve performance so that we can maximize the potential of all employees. I help them to see that they can be a perfect 10 in a perfect job. My job is to get the vision out there, to instill it in each and every person.

I don't have to work hard to bring out the best in people because it's there. All I try and do is enable it to get out. I've learned that the higher you are in the organization, the more you're a servant, and that's okay. I don't want any glory or anything like that. I just want to get the job done and help people to get their jobs done.

Day in and day out, we highlight personal successes, personal accomplishments at every level, and we do that through department meetings. We do that through awards, recognition, notes, prizes, and articles in papers.

I let my leaders do what they know how to do. I find good people doing good things and put a spotlight on them and say you can all learn from these folks. They know what they are doing. They have the heart, the head, and the soul to accomplish the goal. Learn from them.

Our CEO will publicly thank me for my initiative. He is forever working to get me more recognition. There are plenty of opportunities for him to get recognition, and he will have me up front to get the recognition instead.

My job is to make everybody else successful. The exciting part of my job is in the coaching, mentoring, getting people the resources, giving them the recognition, allowing them to be creative, allowing them to run with ideas, having them take responsibility for doing things right, and doing things wrong and learning from them—to create a culture that has people excited about being here.

When I was at St. Vincent's, I brought along a guy. He headed up my floor stripping crew at my previous job. He ended up becoming the assistant director. When I came here, the same thing happened with another employee. I brought him with me from St. Vincent's. He was a natural leader, respected, and his productivity numbers were incredible. After 2 years, we were bumping into each other. A job opened at Southpoint Hospital. I told him about it and told him that he could use me as a reference.

The HR person from Southpoint called, and I told him this person was exceptional. He and another candidate were being considered for the job. I said, "I know who the other guy is, and he is not a leader. He's struggled from hospital to hospital. Take my word for it you want to hire my guy. After I hung up, I heard my employee's phone ring. Shortly after, he came to tell me he had accepted the job. In less than a year, he took over about six departments. He now has about 15 departments, and he's a VP.

One day our administrator was walking down the hall with the administrator from Lakewood. The Lakewood administrator said, "Every time I come in here I get so upset our place is so filthy, we have the worst cleaning scores in the entire Cleveland Clinic Health System." Our administrator told him, "I'm tired of hearing you complain about it. Do something; either make a change or stop complaining."

He got rid of contract cleaning and hired our new assistant director away from us. Since he went over there, Lakewood has actually caught us on patient satisfaction scores and beat us last month. They had a 98% rank, and we had a 97%.

Extended Family

The people who work here understand that taking care of each other is a key element of patient care.

We have always had a culture of quality about our cleaning, but more recently we have developed more of a caring for the patient. We also care about each other. We have a department with people from all over the world, and it is interesting to learn about them, their lives, and their food, just everything. It's all about caring and giving.

I worked at other hospitals, but left to come here because I had heard so much about Fairview. There is a difference in the doctors, the nurses, and the people we work with. They are much friendlier, and we function together as a team. At the other hospitals, there was a much greater divide between doctors and nurses and housekeeping. Here, we are all a team; that is very impressive, and it makes your job so much easier.

I love what I am doing. This community is important to me. We are creating a healthcare system for the next generation.

I want this organization to value caring for each other. I would like to continue to see it relate deeply and be a part of this community. Our people interacting in the community creates who we are as an organization. We need to be out there in the community to share our mission. The clinical stuff we've got. It is the other stuff that is more important to support.

Our work is important, but the most important thing is caring about the people. A couple of Christmases ago I had two single-mom employees, and they were having a difficult time financially. They were hard workers and did the best they could. I thought about these people and went to see our chief administrative officer. I told him the situation and asked him if we had anything at Fairview to help our own people. He said, "I don't think we really do." He told me his dad was coming from Florida for the holidays and always helped families in need at Christmas time. So he said, let me talk to my dad about these two people. He does it anonymously. He came back to me and said his dad was really excited about doing this. He came with his dad and two of his children and picked me up. He is very big on teaching your family to help others. We went to the first house, and they both happened to be there because they were friends. We walked in with huge wicker baskets with turkeys, ham, bread, and all sorts of food. On top of that, he gave them each $300. They didn't know who it was from. That brought me a lot of joy knowing that I was able to help someone.

Afterward the CAO said, "I am sure there are other employees that are in need and not just at the holiday time." He said we ought to work on something like that. Out of that, a group got together and started the Employee Care Fund.

A couple of years ago we were in a United Way Campaign. During the campaign, I realized that we do a lot of fund raising, and it dawned on me that there are a lot of needs right here in our own organization. It occurred to me that we should run our own campaign for each other. So we developed an annual campaign where we raise funds for fellow employees in need. As an example, we have an employee whose husband just lost a job, and they don't have the money for rent or major medical bills. If it has anything to do with health, safety, or welfare, then they can apply for help from the fund. There are certain criteria that are used to evaluate the situation, and if those are met, then it gets approved. That campaign is an incredible example that brought everybody together to take care of each other. It has huge participation. It has great results, and it has created a legacy of sorts.

Being Present

We make a difference in a patient's life everyday, as they do in our lives. Speak and listen to them, and let them know you are there for them and that you care.

My Dad passed away nine years ago, and I like to tell this story about being present. The story is about playing football my freshman year in high school. Nobody goes to those games. There is nobody in the stands. I am on the field, and I am absolutely certain that my dad is there. I didn't think twice about whether or not he was there—my only question was where is he? I looked over at the stands, and there was one guy there. I knew it was him. I didn't think much about it then, but later I thought, "Boy is that important." That presence was something I took for granted when growing up, but it gave me great strength as a person. That is what we do with our staff. We are present.

I was at an event the other day where a nurse's son died unexpectedly right after the holidays. The husband works here, as do several other family members. There was a memorial service. It was really nicely done. It was a packed room. The chaplain asked if anyone would like to share a story, and it was kind of clumsy because no one was prepared for it. No one got up, so I went up and talked to them about how this community is like a family. It is a family when it can support somebody in a time of grief and loss. It was everybody's grief. The organization was acting like a family. It is an important role as a leader to be present at things. Many times it is as important as doing things. That is why people say it is important to round, to manage by walking around. What they are really talking about is being present with your staff. If there are events on the weekend, you need to be here. You support not only the event, but also the people who are doing it.

We have many employees, and my ability to interact with them formally or informally is limited. Rounding is important because it allows me to say who

I am—what counts to me. I think they need to know that their leader shares their values. I like to tell stories about my children, my life experiences, what motivates me, what's important. Doing that allows you to connect out of the business level with an organization, but at a personal level and a relationship level, and that's natural to me.

The chief administrative officer and the chief operating officer have lunch with a small group of staff people once a week. "I have seen the trust level from the informal communication rise. When you have trust, you get engagement. When engagement happens, you get ideas offered to you that make sense."

Leadership Sets the Tone

I value credibility, integrity, and trust. Integrity is doing the right thing. Credibility is doing what you say you are going to do. The two together create trust. Communication is key.

I've got the best job in the world because we have the best people, and I get to watch them do what they do. When they want advice, I give it; sometimes I give it when they don't want it, but I really see my role as facilitating great success by great people who know what they are doing and just want to be able to be allowed to do it.

It is really important to keep your energy up. That is all about motivation. We have to sustain a state of readiness. It has to be satisfying to people, and they have to feel appreciated. Help them to recognize how important the work they are doing really is. Spotlight great leaders, and encourage others to imitate them.

One lady really understands and I'm excited for her because she doesn't need me as a manager anymore. She's doing her job and finding fulfillment in it. She's getting reinforcement with all of these letters and cards that she's making a difference in other people's lives. She's got it. I want to get other people to go from having to do it to seeing how it touches people's lives. That's my goal, so they don't need to be managed and they leave here every day getting it.

When I got a call from the Cleveland Clinic that we had won the Cleveland Clinic World Class Service Award, I had no idea what it was. The lady on the phone told me who she was and I remembered that she used to be a secretary in administration. She told me they wanted to send in a film crew, and I had to be at this banquet. I said, "Wait, wait, wait. If you are sending a film crew in and this is just about me, then don't bother; I am not going to accept the award." She told me I didn't have a choice. I had to show up. I said, "I am not going to come, and I am not going to accept the award. This isn't about me. This is about the department. I didn't do that; they did. So if you want to come in, you can take a picture of the department. Believe me, they won the award. We win it together, or I don't accept it."

The crew came in, and she said, "How about 10 employees?" I said, "How about 30?" She said, "20." So we squeezed 20 employees into the picture. If I had more time, I would have gotten a bus and had them all march across the stage to accept the award. That was big for them.

The World Class Service Award from the Cleveland Clinic was presented to our department. Of all of the recognition the employees received, the director at Lakewood said it the best when he explained, "You know how the Yankees are always good and always in the pennant race? You guys are the Yankees." He had me in tears because I knew the employees understood what he was saying. We have always tried to tell them how much administration appreciates them, but I think he really got to them. That was meaningful for me because I want them to know how valuable they are.

I want my people to leave here satisfied all of the time. Yes, a nice paycheck helps. They have to have a certain level of pay, and I wish I could get them more. They say they are only housekeepers. I ask them if they think the nurses leave here satisfied, and they say yes until I tell them that the nurses don't think the doctors treat them right. I ask them if they think the doctors leave here satisfied, and they say yes until I tell them that the doctors don't think the administration is treating them right. I tell them that satisfaction comes from touching the hearts and lives of others. When you do that, you will leave here every day satisfied thinking, "Wow. I made a difference in someone's life."

Best in Nation

We have a vision. We talk about pretty simple things that are easy for many to understand. We talk about what we want to be. We want to be the best place to work, the best place to receive care, and the best place for our doctors to practice medicine.

We have a big job to do here in keeping the whole hospital clean. We have fewer people to clean even more square footage, and we always have a sense of urgency; so, we work to take care of things in the right way. It all started because I developed a welcome card to go in the patient rooms to let the patients know that our goal in Environmental Services is to be the best in the nation. We not only want to meet their expectations but also want to exceed their expectations.

What followed was the Road Map to Success and the GO MAD Program. The GO MAD (Go Make A Difference) program links directly to the Fairview vision. Each Environmental Services employee is given a MAD Sheet with three questions to fill in: (1) Today I made a difference in a patient or visitor's life by (Best Place to Receive Care). (2) Today I made a difference in an employee's life by (Best Place To Work). (3) Today I made a difference in a physician's life by (Best Place to Practice Medicine).

We decided that we needed a welcome card in the room that said our goal was to exceed their expectations. I thought this may drop our scores because now we have to live up to what we say on the card. We thought about it for a couple of days and realized we had to get the employees involved or else we would fail. That is how we came up with some of the ideas. We want complaints so that we can make it right. Then we asked, "What could we do that truly exceeds their expectations, to make our patients say, 'Wow, I never expected that.'" It has to be something that has meaning to the patient. There are lots of things we can do, but if it doesn't have meaning, then it is a waste.

One of the things we decided to do was to check back with the patients before the employees went home for the day. I thought the employees would like it, and it would make their day more exciting. This is our 2:55 checkout. This is a mandatory program where the housekeepers go back into each patient room and say, "It is getting close to the end of my shift and I just wanted to check back and see if there was anything more I could do for you. I have the time."

Then we did the newspaper. We learned about one of our employees who was buying newspapers for her patients. She was actually going down herself buying eight newspapers every day. This is a woman who doesn't make a lot of money, and she wouldn't let us pay her back. Patients were so happy about it that we decided as a department to do it for every patient.

We added silk flowers in the rooms. One day, while doing rounds, I noticed that some patients didn't have any flowers in their room. So, I decided, "Why not cheer up the room just that little bit more and put a little flower arrangement in their room?" Since not all patients receive flowers while they are in the hospital, we decided to put flowers in each room. We had arrangements of silk flowers prepared, and we placed them in containers and glued them in place. With each arrangement is a laminated card that says, "These flowers are for your enjoyment during your stay at Fairview. Please do not remove the flowers so that the next patient can enjoy them also. Thank you (Courtesy of Environmental Services)." They are even in the public restrooms.

We scripted the 2:55 checkout. It went well for most of the employees, and they got on board with it. In initiating this change, we had to do one thing at a time. You don't want to overwhelm people. It took four months to get 80% of the employees on board. We sent thank you cards to the homes of the employees who were doing it right 100% of the time. Then we had a meeting where we told everyone that we needed 100% commitment to the program from 100% of the employees 100% of the time. If we are going to be the best, we need everyone on board, and we will help those who need it; however, it is mandatory. Why? Because we want you to be successful, and we want you to have a great evaluation. We believe that once you start doing this you are going to enjoy your work more and feel better when you leave. Then we started holding the supervisors accountable, which in turn meant that they started holding the employees accountable. Once new employees come on board and recognize that this is part of their responsibilities, then it is easy.

After about a year of posting our patient satisfaction scores, 8 or 10 employees came to me and said we really don't care about how we are scoring against the other Cleveland clinic hospitals. Where are we nationally? You say we want to be best in the nation. We already know we are the best in the clinic system. Where are we nationally? It was then that I realized that they got it; they really understood what we were trying to do.

The staff satisfaction has increased, and they don't feel like just housekeepers anymore. They now feel like an integral part of the process. Along with the staff satisfaction came the patient satisfaction improvements. These people are very proud of their hospital.

One of the questions on the patient survey is this: "Did they exceed your expectations?" We have always been pushing that as our goal because we have had successful survey results, but we took it one step further. Instead of worrying about our vision to be the best in the Cleveland Clinic System, no, let's go bigger than that. Let's try to go for being the best in the nation. Not everybody has the opportunity to be a movie star or an NBA player, but if you work in our department, you have an opportunity to be a part of something great because we are going to be the best in the nation. That's how I came up with the welcome card, and we started thinking, "What are we going to do to really exceed their expectations?"

One of the housekeepers buys reading glasses and has a bunch of them on her cart because a lot of patients forget to bring their reading glasses. So if she sees someone struggling to read, she gives him or her a pair. She doesn't ask to get paid, she just gives them to the patient.

One lady sings to her patients. We have an environmental services employee known to many patients as the "singing housekeeper." She uses her talent to comfort and cheer patients.

When we see someone who is hopelessly lost in the hospital, our people don't point him or her in the general direction. Rather, they walk them down the hall to their intended destination.

We have an evening housekeeper in ICU who makes origami birds for everybody. All of the patients at night talk about these origami birds and the lady that makes them. She's like this famous person.

We have a system on our computer that tracks when a patient is discharged and alerts the housekeeper by means of a pager. I'm really excited about this process, and my numbers show that we can turn a bed over quickly once we know and identify it. The problem is that it took 91 minutes before Environmental Services was ever notified. Once we were notified, we turned the beds over in about 40 minutes. We ended up putting our own system in place. The transport volunteers call when they take the patient out of the room. That call sets off our pager, and the information is entered into the computer system. Anybody can look at the data. Our turnaround time on the dayshift is now under 25 minutes, whereas the national average is 96 minutes.

As a manager in the hospital I am accountable to write two thank you cards per week. Because I have 100+ employees, two cards a week doesn't go very far. I realized that by including my supervisors and leads in writing cards we could reach many more people. We discuss all of the employees—not only in our department, but also in other departments.

Instead of just sending two thank you cards, I usually send out four; then I'm exceeding expectations. My goal is to exceed expectations. I'm trying to develop the managers working for me to go beyond just sending a card that says, "Thanks, good job." A good example would be bed tracking. For about four months, most of our cards focused on bed tracking. The card would say, "You know our turnover goal is 30 minutes or less. If we want to exceed expectations, we will need to get down to 25 minutes, and I believe you have the ability to excel. You went from 50 down to 42, and you were at 60 the month before. So I have great confidence that you will be able to get to 25 minutes and exceed expectations." So we try to always take the reward and recognition and streamline it back to what we are trying to achieve. We are always trying to connect the dots. This way most of our employees get about eight cards a year. Last year I think we averaged 6.7 cards per person. Even with low performers we try to find something that they are doing right to try to build on.

One example involves an employee named Josephine. We started a patient callback system here at the hospital, and I noticed that her name was constantly being mentioned. Usually the housekeeper is mentioned in a lot of them, but she is always mentioned by name. So I told her that it was intriguing that out of 27 times we were mentioned in two weeks her name was mentioned 13 times. She's definitely doing something over and above what we are scripting.

I asked her to sit down and talk with me so that we could learn from her and improve our process. It was obvious that she had figured out how to modify her script to make it personal. She told me, "Well, I just tell them that my name is Josephine, and I try to make it personal like that's a big J, Josephine, capital J, and I'm going to go write my name on the board over here and I'm going to put a smile here because my day is to make your day. I want to let you know that if you need anything I'm around on this unit. You just let the nurse know that you need to see Josie, and Josie will take good care of you."

So, she constantly reinforces her name three or four times. She walks up to them, makes eye contact, and listens to them speak back to her. She says she tries to get her name in four times—writes it on the board, a big J with a smile. She also learns their names. She will remember their name because during rounds, I have heard her say, "Oh, I want you to meet so and so." She has the ability to remember people's names, and I think that helps a lot too. She does an incredible job, and we are now using her to train new employees.

Touching Lives and Hearts

Our badges say Environmental Services, but we are about much more than keeping clean.

Interaction with patients is encouraged.

The staff used to feel that they had to be invisible—that they were only the housekeepers. Now they go into the room and introduce themselves and ask permission to clean the room, and before they leave, they ask if there is anything else I can do. I have the time. This has greatly improved the staff's job satisfaction. There are great stories about patient comments.

It is job satisfaction, too. You feel so much better when you help somebody. On a daily basis, you can see how fortunate you are as a person, and the spirituality here is unbelievable. I have been a catholic all of my life, but I never really understood spirituality until I came here.

If I were sick, this is where I would want to be.

I handle the lost and found for the hospital. A lot of times older folks forget things and have no way to come and pick up their items. So a lot of times I will drop stuff off on my way home. One time I dropped of some stuff at an apartment, and the lady and her husband insisted that I come in, sit down, and talk to them. They were so sweet, and she gave me this huge bag of tomatoes. She wanted me to stay there forever. They were so grateful that I brought the clothes to them, and they just wanted somebody to talk to. Then on top of that, they sent me a thank you card.

One of our staff, who has a perpetual smile, had a hard time with the implementation of the end-of-day checkout program. We told her that it wasn't optional but, rather, that it was mandatory. In the fifth room she went to, she asked if there was anything she could do for the person before she went home because she had the time. The patient said, "Yes, I could really use a hug." She gave the patient a hug, and the patient cried. Two rooms later she approached a patient who appeared to be sleeping and the wife of the patient asked if there was something she needed. She explained the greeting program to her. The wife said, "My husband is dying of cancer, and he isn't very responsive right now; I could sure use a hug." She came out of the room crying and shared the story with us. It showed her the impact she was having in just one day. That got shared throughout the hospital. It set the program off. It gave the whole program a really big jump in the department. This employee has been here for 25 years. If she only cleaned one room a day, she would have cleaned 109,000 patient rooms. Up until recently, there were two patients in a room. That amounts to 218,000 lives she has touched. If four people did that, you could touch every life in the city of Cleveland.

One of our housekeepers told me about this patient who was really irate. She was really mad at the nurse taking care of her. So our housekeeper took her aside and said, "Can we go talk quietly?" They sat down in her room and she said, "I know you're upset with this nurse. You probably have valid reasons, but please don't feel like everybody is like that. We really care about people." To make the nurse look better, she suggested, "Maybe the nurse is having a rough day. That's not an excuse if her behavior was not appropriate, but everybody has bad days. I'm here for you. Is there anything you need? There are many people in this hospital that will do anything for you." She went on, "Did you ever have a foot massage?"

The patient said, "No."

"I'm going to give you a foot massage."

This story just blew me away. That patient forgot everything because our housekeeper did that. Our housekeeper had never given anybody a foot massage before, but she gave this patient one.

We had a cancer patient who was here off and on for a couple of years for treatment. She was in my area the last 2 weeks of her life. I didn't realize she was dying until we talked. We became pretty close during that time. We shared a lot. We prayed a lot. We cried a lot. I got to know her family, her husband, her mother, and her father. One of her requests was to get married to the father of her children before she passed away. They had been together about 25 years.

It was pretty comical what happened on her wedding day. Hospice, several nurses, and the singing housekeeper were all involved. Two days later the wedding took place. The future husband had trouble finding a notary public, and we had everybody trying to find one. Eventually we found one. The husband had to go downtown, get the marriage license, and get it signed and notarized and come back. In the meantime, we were getting things ready in the atrium for the wedding. On his way back, he realized that he had forgotten the rings and had to go back home to get the rings. The wedding was scheduled for 5:00 p.m. but really took place at 7:30 p.m. Their pastor escorted him home to get the ring and back to make sure that nothing else happened. Then we couldn't find the bride because one of the family members had rolled her down somewhere, and they were supposed to come back. We finally found her, and they had cut back on her morphine so that she could say her vows. Somehow it all worked, and 3 days later she passed away. It took a lot of work from a lot of people, but that was a wish come true for our patient. It proved that by working together as a team we could accomplish something for our patient.

Ministry of Caring

When we are not doing well, it is because we are not connecting to the mission of the people. Their personal mission, not the organizational mission. It is their personal mission that we mess up on.

Your job is to do the professional things you are hired for, but your job is also to support each other because the best place to work is the connection between each of us. It is not the connection between a program or a service or facility or some technology. That is the goal.

Two ladies had a problem with each other. I sat down with them and we talked. I helped them each realize the other person's intent was not to hurt their feelings. It was just that people from different backgrounds and different cultures view things in a different way. Well, to make a long story short, these two people ended up apologizing to one another, hugging each other. I found out later that the one girl actually went out and bought the other person a little gift just to say how sorry she was for hurting her and now they're good friends.

Management is here to help us. Their vision, their approach, is good. They are like the good shepherd. Because they are good, then we are good.

We do the state of the organization for our leaders and for our medical staff. I talked about the business of the region, the direction, and the priorities—where the organization has gone and where it can go—but then pulled them back and said, "In order for us to go in that direction, you have to take a moment and ask yourself, 'Why did I join the ministry of healthcare?' That's a very personal question. It is individual to each of us." I said, "When you find that why, you're going to find your own mission." I was trying to get them to think about it because too often they think about all of the sound and fury that's health care and not about the core of health care. I suggested to them that all of what we're talking about for the next year really means little unless you can connect your mission to this organization's mission and direction. That resonated and connected in an audience of doctors and my direct leaders, in the organization. I believe that we spend way too much time talking about organization's mission and not the individual mission of people and whether we are living up to that individual mission by the way we conduct an organization. That also calls them to do the same thing with folks that they lead and I talked about that a little.

As you lead, you have to find that personal mission and pull that out in folks that you lead and be true to that. I said, "It's very simple to define what we say as our vision goal—best place to work, best place to practice medicine, and the best place to receive care." I said, "If you think about it and do this regularly folks, what's the best place that you worked before you came here?" I will tell people to just go back in their mind, take time to do that. They won't think about a building, a care process, or equipment; they are going to think about people. They are going to think about the friends that they worked with that supported them professionally and personally. They are going to think about people who had a mission and whether the organization connected to it and allowed them to do it. That's what they need to do on a daily basis as opposed to all of the to-do lists of a business plan. It won't happen if they do it that way.

If you don't connect to the soul of the individual when you're leading, you are just going to lead them into the wilderness. You are not going to achieve their goal or the organization's goal.

One example was when marketing was doing focus group research. I went and listened to former patients and families of patients talk about Fairview Hospital. The discussions were so positive that I thought everybody at Fairview should hear those comments. I asked the marketing people and the focus group people to give me the live audio of everything. We made a DVD and sent it to every employee and medical staff here. We did about 4,000 of them with a personal letter saying, "This is what happened here, and you need to hear what people are saying about us." We sent it home so that they could play it for themselves and for their family and so that they could be proud of the place. That is an example of how we acknowledge our people and reinforce our Service Excellence Program. In those comments, it's not that the doctor took out the right thing. They are as follows: "Somebody was kind to me." "Somebody sat on my bed at 2:00 in the morning and held my hand." "My place was clean." "The food was good." "Somebody gave me directions." "They walked me down the hall." These were all courtesy, respect,

dignity issues that any one of us wants. Our whole focus of our patient satisfaction and employee and doctor satisfaction is these things. If you take it
from the other side of the conversation, it really is true; this is the really
important stuff that our patients or the family members are talking about.
This affirms why we really are the benchmark for the best patient satisfaction
in the Cleveland Clinic Health System.

Accountability

Our director of Environmental Services is such a visionary. He is systematic.
He has heart. He gets it across to the employees. He is the only person I know
who can fire somebody for cause and have him or her thank him. I know why.
He clearly explains his expectations to them. He keeps track of them. If they
are not meeting expectations, he tells them, "Here is your improvement plan.
If you don't meet this, I have to let you go." If they don't meet it, he has a final
exit interview and says, "You know we worked through this." They say, "I
know I didn't make the plan. I appreciate your helping me understand where
I have my faults. In my next job, I am going to work on that extra hard." He
is able to do that. He has a system with check sheets for the employees, and it
all rolls into their evaluation. It is exactly the way it is supposed to be. All of
his employees love him because nothing he asks of them is unexpected.

We used to have level pay—for example, all the housekeepers got paid the
same. Now we have pay for performance, and it is much better.

We pay close attention to the survey scores, and employees are accountable for
those scores: 100% commitment by 100% of the employees 100% of the
time. This includes floaters—holding people accountable for the report card
or scorecard. This system keeps us as managers from being inconsistent. These
report cards tie into their evaluations and in turn to their pay for performance. This includes holding our supervisors accountable for doing their jobs
as well. Everyone within our department is held accountable for the things for
which they are responsible. Everyone knows that we provide them with the
details of what they have to do, and if they do those things, they will be successful. There are no gray areas.

Housekeeping created accountability when they stopped their staff before the
end of the shift and had them go back into the patient rooms to ask if there is
anything more they could do for the patient. That owns the job! They really
get it. This is as smart as I have ever seen. It creates great satisfaction for

patients and staff alike. The staff member becomes accountable not to house-keeping but to the patient. That is what I think is remarkable. The patient motivates the staff daily. They thank them. They appreciate them. Housekeeping gave them a way to do their job that happens beautifully and naturally.

I know that we have a system that works, and you can hold people account-able. We have had the highest employee satisfaction scores for five years, the highest physician satisfaction scores, and the highest patient satisfaction scores. The probability of that happening is one out of something like 600,000. It doesn't happen by chance. It's a lot of hard work. It can be done in every department if you implement the tools we use.

Voices of the Patients

The housekeeper was outstanding. She talked with me everyday and truly cared about me. She was so nice to my grandson and really improved my health by creating a happy environment. She is a special person.

Housekeeping was excellent because they would sit and talk with me. They were always trying to make sure everyone was happy. They got me the paper early every day, which was a big deal to me.

I really appreciated the housekeeper I had on Sunday. She went and bought me a paper. That was so nice of her. I felt as if I were in a hotel.

A staff member went to the cafeteria and got me a salad when the dinner tray wasn't very good.

The CEO got a puzzle book for me when I was in the hospital.

I felt good when the staff took the time to pray with me.

The housekeeper rubbed my legs with lotion after her shift.

The housekeeper was wonderful. I think she does a better job of making peo-ple feel better than the doctors do. Also, the nurse was very good. She is very calm and does a great job of answering my questions.

Heart and Soul of Housekeeping

In our department, it's much more than just cleaning. We do greetings at the end of the day, going from patient room to patient room.

We are considered a part of the team. We are more than just the invisible housekeepers, and we help them whenever they need it. There are many times when they will ask us to help them boost up the patient. We always ask them if there is anything we can do to help. Now we have the GO MAD Program that formalizes what many of us had been doing all along. It really helps the new housekeepers to become more assertive and communicative.

We really like our jobs so much that we have a lot of longevity in the group.

The joyfulness is in my patients. I love to make them smile and forget for maybe just a little while where they are and what they are facing.

I like talking with the patients because I know that a lot of them are going through difficult times.

I have to say I feel contentment and joy, and I know I do a good job. I think it's because I take pride in my work, my job cleaning, and my floor. I have moms and dads thank me for a good cleaning job well done.

Whether it is greeting patients each morning, delivering the paper, or doing our 2:55 checkout, we say kind things just to see our patients smile or laugh. To do something special for them makes a whole lot of difference to me. It makes me feel good to have changed someone's life around. It's the little things we do for the patients that makes a job well done.

The head nurses along with several helpers were organizing the move of the patients to a new unit. Everyone was full of anticipation. It reminded me of Christmas Eve when I was a little girl. I could not wait until the last of the patients were moved so I could get started in the new unit. I have to say that I wake up every day and I still feel excited to get to work and be in such a beautiful surrounding.

I work in Pediatrics. Five years ago I went into a room and was dusting off the TV, and I heard this little voice saying thank you for dusting off my TV so I can see better. His name was Adam, and he was not quite two years old.

I feel important because I do other things to help people besides just cleaning. Sometimes I feel that since I work in the ER I can help in many other ways, and that's what I like about where I work.

A few months ago I had an overweight patient; she was always feeling down. I would come in every morning and ask her how was she. Some days she would say nothing. One day she said she didn't feel pretty. She said that her hair was a mess, and she did not have her makeup. I told her that if she wanted I could do her hair. Do you know what? She said, "Okay." I took a brush and did her hair, and I polished her nails. She looked in the mirror and smiled. I made her day.

There was a time when I went in a room and my son's coach was a patient. He didn't know that I worked here and was impressed with my work and wrote out a star card. He made me feel good and comfortable in the way I treated him. He also told the nurses about how my job performance was. This made me feel good about what I do and inspired me to do even more.

I walked into a patient's room, and she was crying. She told me she had cancer and was waiting for the doctor to come and see her. She told me she didn't have much time left. I hugged her. I told her we all only have today. I tried to comfort her with words. By the time I left her room, she was smiling. I thought I made a big difference in her thinking for the moment.

I recall a patient on my floor who was very unhappy about being in the hospital for the holidays. I came in to do my daily cleaning and found myself engaged in a conversation with this patient. All it took was a little attention and listening to him to brighten his day. As I do my work on a daily basis, I meet and greet people everyday and walk away with a smile.

There was a patient in room 312 that had been there for several days. She was getting ready to be discharged when she told me that she was going outside to smoke. When she came back, she surprised me with a gift. She said that she appreciated all of the things I had done for her.

I was cleaning a patient's room and had finished mopping the floor. I told the man not to walk on the floor for 10 minutes because he might slip and fall. The man looked at me and said, "I won't be getting up without my leg." I looked over, and the man's leg was leaning against the wall. I was speechless.

He started to laugh, and it made me feel less embarrassed. We began to talk and discovered we were both diabetics.

I can recall when the skilled nursing unit had a patient who was 91 years old. We held hands and told each that we would never forget one another. She always wanted me to stay in the room and never leave her. She was discharged, and we said our goodbyes. As I left the room, I started to cry. This sweet lady touched my heart in so many ways.

I want to say that the patients are what make my job so joyful. I enter the room with a smile. I like speaking to the patient as I'm cleaning the room. Some of the patients I joke and kid with and make them laugh and smile. When a patient laughs and smiles, it makes me feel good about what I do here at Fairview Hospital. There are patients that are very ill, so I just comfort them.

When I've had a rough day, I go to my director's office. He buys me a cup of coffee and talks to me until I feel good enough to return to my work.

I admire both my director and assistant director in Environmental Services because I know somewhat of their humble beginnings. They've not only shown us how leaders are born but have invested in our lives as well. They encourage us to be truly the best that we can be. Truly, they walked their talk—that's why they are such effective leaders in our department. I'm proud to be a part of their team. This is one of the reasons this hospital is the best place to work, receive care, and practice medicine.

I admire two wonderful people: my director and assistant director. This is a short story to show you how our department pulls together like they are family. About three years ago I was in need of a good friend who would just listen to me. I had no one to turn to until my director and assistant director told me the door is always open. I took them up on their offer in November. I walked down the hall wondering what could they possible say to me. Could they really care? When I walked into their office they greeted me with a warm smile and a gentle hug. I told them what a difficult time I was having. Christmas was coming up. I am a single mother. I could not afford anything for my son—not even a good meal. On Christmas day, to my surprise, my CAO and assistant director were at my door with a basket full of unbelievable things. I cried. That was the best Christmas ever.

Editor Commentary

The senior leaders at the Cleveland Clinic and of the Fairview organization have embarked on a journey to service excellence. They have established the right path, given the right messages, and supported the departmental leadership in environmental services. Through the departmental leaders— in particular the director and the assistant director—the vision becomes reality each day. It's their audacious, bold goal of being the best housekeeping department in the country that has transformed the department.

Once they set this goal, the leaders worked to accomplish it through an unyielding focus on believing in their employees and helping the employees, in turn, to believe and have confidence in themselves. "The best is already there (within the employee)" is a guiding management belief. The departmental leaders believe in their employees, their capabilities, and their talents; they are committed to maximizing (and appreciating) what each one of them brings to the table. Their philosophy of connecting to each employee's individual mission has had a powerful impact. The effect on the employees, as told in stories, has been as transformative for them as it has been on the patients, families, and nurses who are their customers. The passion and dedication of the leaders to make their staff successful is extraordinary.

The departmental leaders have made significant investments in having good processes—selecting/hiring the right people, excellent training and coaching, and unassailable accountability. They have also implemented creative ideas like the 2:55 p.m. checkout. More important than all of this, however, is the pride that they have instilled in their department. The employees always made a difference— they know it, feel it, and talk about it. We all need to know we make a difference—clearly these men and women do. Whereas they used to view themselves "as just housekeepers," they now see how important they are to the whole team.

The commitment on the part of the leaders to also recognize the unique personal and financial circumstances that some of their employees are faced with is apparent. The actions of leaders to support their employees who are having a hard time—whether through individual acts of charity or putting together the Employee Charity Fund—these actions speak at least as loudly as their words. They are present for their staff in both big and little moments. They take action to support their team.

This isn't just about being nice to their employees, however—they make their expectations very clear and hold their staff accountable for this high level of performance. They have confidence in their employee's abilities and because of that set high expectations for them. This makes it possible to the environmental services department at Fairview Hospital to achieve even greater goals than the staff had ever dreamed were possible. They are proud of their efforts and success, and it shows.

Table 7-1 Organizational Demographics

Organization	Geisinger Health System
Location	Danville, PA
Setting	Rural
Communities served	Rural
Type of organization	Health system (3 hospitals plus a children's hospital, a large group practice, 41 community practice sites, a chemical dependency treatment facility, and an HMO)
Number of beds	866
Number of FTEs	10,000
Scope of service	Primary care, specialty care, and tertiary and quaternary care
Organizational awards	Solucient 100 Top Hospitals 2005
	Most Wired 2006
Focus area	Geisinger Medical Group (GMG)—Dermatology
Focus area served	Patients—25,000/year
	Residents/fellows 10
	Students—approximately 20 per year
Best practice	*GMG dermatology is currently at the 99th percentile in Press Ganey's Medical Practice database.*

A Culture of Coaching and Developing Others

Contributor: Susan O. Wood

The stories in this chapter are the voices of the senior executive team at Geisinger Health System, the medical director and nurse manager for the dermatology clinic, the senior director for guest services, physicians and staff members from the dermatology clinic, their patients, and members of the community. Here are their stories.

GEISINGER HEALTH SYSTEM

Role Model

The physician director says, "If you see me as a patient, you are my responsibility."

"It starts in this department with the top," says a nurse. The director remembers the patient's name, his or her family, and his or her past. He will see any patient that needs to be seen. He goes to their house or nursing home on weekends and at night. He's a legend. Everyone underneath him emulates him.

He instills values in other people. We always see patients, no matter what. If the patient asks if they can come in on Tuesday, he says, "Of course." He expects us to do the same and acknowledges all of us for doing this.

If somebody walks in and says, "I need to be seen now," we find somebody to see them. "No" is not part of the vocabulary. It's just great.

I absorb as much as possible from him. How does he remember patients' names, their children, and what they are doing? I want to have the relationship with the patient that he has.

We like to talk about the fact that we are so productive yet everybody gets along so well. That is extremely unique. We often try and figure out our director's management style and why it is that he's been so unbelievably effective. I used to believe that in order to be the head of a productive department that you had to be somewhat of what I used to call "malignant." You had to have a dark side. I don't believe that anymore. I have never seen a department like this before, and I've never seen a leader like our physician director. I don't know how you would ever duplicate it. He carefully picks the people that he chooses to work for him, and then he really leads by example: which is highly effective. I think you have to have the right followers, and I think you have to be careful about who you pick.

I've only been here for 2 ½ years. The physician director's attitude is instilled in other people. It is not always the most efficient practice, but one that is very high in patient satisfaction. First off, we always see patients no matter what. I had a patient call me a week before her appointment was coming up, and she said, "Gosh, I got into neurology on Tuesday. Is there any way that I can come back and see you when I get there that day?" "Of course" is the answer. I learned this from our director because he will see patients at the drop of a hat. He will ask how patients are doing if he sees them in the grocery store. "How are you doing, Mrs. Smith? How's that ulcer?" Around here, people will show you things in the grocery store. He doesn't bat an eyelash. The rest of the clinic functions that way because he has trained us all, whether we know it or not.

One of the surgeons has such a wonderful bedside manner. It always amazes me. These people are getting disfiguring surgeries on their face, and he has this way of making them so calm. He just puts his hands on them and says, "It's going to be okay." I've learned that the laying on of hands is so valuable to patients. Just that simple touch is so reassuring to them, and I think it is rewarding for us as well. So I tried to incorporate that in part of what I do. I'm trying to be a sponge.

I've been real lucky—so many times—to get recognition from patients. That continues to mean something after all of these years. When I was teaching family practice residents, I got a couple of awards from students. My colleagues are generous with acknowledgment. My boss, the chair of psychiatry is very specific about recognizing my efforts. I'm not a physician, and I feel a part of things. I understand the practice. In a workshop one day about teaching residents, a physician said that he'd like to see how I would do it. That was a sense of respect. I felt very good.

Our CEO recognizes special efforts by sending notes. He notices when something you do makes a difference. I recently worked on an event where we were developing relationships in the community that will influence the future course of Geisinger. The CEO wrote a note thanking me for going out of my way to make it successful. The chief medical officer, medical director, and chief nurse executive pay careful attention to recognizing special efforts. I frequently find a fruit tray on the NICU or another unit that the chief nurse executive has delivered to express gratitude for meeting a challenge. Appreciation is part of the culture.

We've got a CEO who engages people in visioning as well as anyone I've ever seen. His ability to create an area of overlap that makes sense to folks, which they can relate to, is superb. It comes out of discussion with a lot of people. He's meeting face to face with thousands of people in the organization. It has made a difference in the organization. We know where we are going. We are doing visioning again for the next five years. That first vision actually came true. Now we are going to the next level. People have great confidence that we can do it. That's really an example when you talk about role modeling.

House Calls

Our doctors always give their home phone numbers out. A patient that had surgery called her physician at home because he was bleeding. He lived in Lewisburg and had no way to get to Geisinger. The physician went to get him because it had to be taken care of right away. She drove to Lewisburg, picked the gentleman up, and brought him to the ER. She took care of the patient's problem and drove him back to his home. He needed to get his mail first, so she took him to get his mail. It was not a big deal to her. Where do you find people that make house calls like that?

There have been times when we nurses have driven patients home in the evening to make sure that they were settled and had everything they needed. We do this especially if they were going home to an empty house and were going to be by themselves.

I had an incident one time at my church where there was a patient that had a leg ulcer. He was concerned that it was getting worse. We called a physician from my church and asked him what to do. He said he would be over to see him tomorrow. He went to his house and made a house call. He did. It's just the most comfortable, caring place that you could want to work.

Last year a second-year resident had a gentleman patient who had psoriasis from head to toe. He was not responding to treatment and went on disability, losing his job in construction. He could have died. This man could not wear shoes or use his hands. The resident tried to get him a new medication, but it was not yet approved. So we had a meeting with all of the physicians and came up with the idea that we needed to get another opinion from one of the nation's experts in this disease. It turns out that there is a rheumatologist/dermatologist only about 3 or 4 hours away in New Brunswick, New Jersey. We called Robert Wood Johnson to make an appointment. I thought this was the right thing to do. We had to do something for him. It was the resident's idea, and I thought this was great. Let's do it.

Our resident and head nurse picked up the patient at home and drove him 2½ hours to New Jersey. The patient got new medication. The patient called on Monday morning and said, "Doc, you are not going to believe this. I got my fingernails back."

"You can't have your fingernails back, that's too quick."

"Well, I'm going to come up later this week and show you," and he did. That medicine absolutely turned his life around. He was close to death's door several times, and with one infusion over a weekend, he improved dramatically.

The director stopped by a nursing home to visit a patient. It was getting to hard for her to come into the clinic. He said, "And at the end, we are going to sit down and watch Jeopardy together."

A physician got alarming lab results on a patient. He called the patient and the line was busy. Realizing that the patient may be in trouble, he drove to her house to check on her.

Part of the message with house calls is that patients live in their world, not ours. How can they do as well as possible? We need to consider what their world is and venture into it more than what our standard thinking is.

Patients First

This is not a hotel service approach. We focus on partnering with the patient. The patients that come here see a real difference in their relationships with all the professionals here. They see themselves having a type of partnership that makes them accountable and proud to be getting better because they are a part of the decisions.

Our patients, all of our patients, are very special to us. We like to treat our patients the way that we would like to be treated or that we would like a family member to be treated. Our patients are number one. Like she said, that's the whole reason we're here. If we didn't have our patients, we wouldn't be here.

I see every complaint and all patient-satisfaction feedback. The complaints are a little job. When we get them, I call the patient. They are astounded. It creates a positive relationship.

I try to convey that I respect the patient immediately. Older people need special advocacy. Yesterday I had a woman—83 years old. She came in with her 90-year-old husband. She had seen at least a dozen physicians over 10 years and had inappropriate treatment for skin cancer. It was a huge mess. These people can get so lost and need someone to help them navigate the system. Somebody has to help them. So I promised them that the phone calls would be made and that they would get to the right people.

Patient perceptions are critical. It is good that top leadership is focused on health outcomes and measurement. Financial measures count, but most important is the patient perception of their experience and how the patient perception relates to outcomes. There is pressure to move people in and out of the hospital, and even change rooms and beds—degrading the quality of their experience. We know that there is a price for moving patients. It's more than financial measures that count here. It's a combination of leadership, focus, and measurement. I'm satisfied with that—I'm excited. It's the way it should be.

Just two weeks ago, one of the desk receptionists noticed that a patient who was signing in was extremely anxious. So she came and got me and said, "This woman is scared to death about her surgery and is just so anxious that she can hardly talk." I went out to see what was going on. I could see that the woman was really anxious so I told her surgeon.

I said to him, "You know, your next patient for surgery is so anxious. Could you go talk to her?"

He went out in the waiting room and took her hand and said, "I understand you are worried about this surgery." He spent 10 minutes with her just talking about what was going to happen and what to expect. It made all the difference in the world.

She went up to the desk person three times and said, "I have never been in a department that would do that." She felt so much better. The desk receptionist immediately picked up on the fact that this woman was anxious and didn't just think, "Oh, she's anxious." Instead she thought, "I need to fix this." Those are everyday occurrences in this department. It's a joy to work here.

The dermatology department secretary demonstrates thorough, efficient completion of all tasks. She is a friendly, compassionate, and perspicacious person. She is aware of people's feelings and needs. For example, she overheard an older gentleman say that he had left belongings in another clinic. It was late in the day. Quietly she went to the clinic and retrieved his belongings. This allowed him to leave the hospital directly from dermatology. People like her make our department run smooth and seamless. Harmony is maintained.

There was a patient that was being seen for surgery. I'm a receptionist, and I was making a return appointment for her. She said to her husband that he had a mark on his lip and that he should get it checked. He said, "Oh, I just cut that shaving. It's not a problem."

I made her appointment and then said, "Would you like me to see if I can get one of the doctors to take a look at it? It will only take a minute."

He didn't really want to but said, "Okay."

I went back to the doctors and told them their patient's husband wants something checked. They said, "Sure. We'll take a look at it." It turned out to be a skin cancer. When he came in later for his appointment, he gave me a hug.

As a receptionist, my job is so much easier because of the team that I have behind me. Our doctors are so good that when we ask them something, even if they are busy, they will take time out to talk to a patient. They may not be able to do surgery or a full appointment on that day, but they do know whether it's something we should take care of soon. That just gives such a good rapport with our patients. Sometimes they do have to wait to get signed in, but they are not irate. Our doctors do not rush them through, no matter how busy they are. If somebody comes in on a wrong appointment and if there is anyone available, we do not turn him or her away. I've been here for six years, and I do not remember turning somebody away unhappy because they weren't seen.

If there is somebody out in the waiting room that you know is hesitant about their appointment, we ask them if they want coffee or a cookie. We'll do anything to make them feel a little better. We used to have little things at our desk that said, "The patient always comes first." We also have birthday stickers for patients. If it's their birthday, we put a sticker with their paper. So, we can give them a sticker and wish them a happy birthday.

There was one surgical patient. When I scheduled this patient I could hear the anxiety in her voice. She was scheduled out a few weeks. I ended up calling her back and said, "The only reason I'm calling is because I could hear that there was some anxiety. I just wanted to reassure you that this isn't going to worsen for you in the meantime and. . . ." Do you know, when the patient came in for her appointment, it was around the same time that my daughter was ill. She came in to meet me. I wasn't at work because of my daughter's illness. I got a note from her. She ended up bringing in a prayer for my daughter. It just goes to show you that we are all in this world together.

Patients here are so appreciative. I left for a fellowship for two years. When I returned, former patients came back. So many gave me a hug and were glad to see me, saying, "I waited to book an appointment with you." I pray for guidance every day and to give time and consideration they deserve.

I came to Danville for a residency interview. I drove into town and said to myself, "This is not happening—no way." I came to the clinic to see patients. I knew nothing about Geisinger. As I was driving away, I called my husband and said, "This is where I want to be." I was floored by the way patients were treated. After a few minutes with Vic, I would see these people come to life. He put his hands on them. "How are you doing?" He would listen to them. It was therapeutic. The respect for patients is unique. This place is phenomenal. The staff here is top notch. I would bring my family here.

All 600 physicians at Geisinger get individual scores on patient satisfaction. Everybody knows his or her own scores. They know it matters, and they want to get scores that reflect good relationships with patients. Dermatology is a department that does superbly well at this. All of their physician scores are high. They are at the 99th percentile, reflecting how they put patients first. Last week a physician in another department came in to talk about scores for him and two colleagues, as they had dropped. They raised a challenge to scoring. "The data have to be wrong. If my colleague has to go to one of these coaching sessions, he will quit." I was aware of how angry he was, but I know that the data are the data. Not every physician agrees with how we are using the data; however, every physician knows what his or her patient satisfaction score is, and they know it matters. That is one of the strong positive things. If nobody used the data, I wouldn't get calls like that.

The real goal is that we want loyalty to the patients because we are serving them so well. This is part of good care. The numbers reflect the best way we can get a handle on it.

Shared Vision

We have just gone through a visioning exercise where 6,000 of our 11,000 employees told us what they think the goals should be for the next five years. Now that we are doing well, how do we want to use that robust operation? What do we want to do that's particularly appropriate to our anatomy and our background? Our mission? What can we do that might differentiate us from everybody else in the country?

There were as many administrative clerks and radiology technicians as there were doctors. Twenty-five key words on signs had been given to people: loyalty, perseverance, communication, and resilience. We needed to discuss how these values apply to our goals for the next five years.

It was the most amazing 3½ hours I had ever sat through—absolutely energizing. People had remarkable and creative things to say, and it showed me that if you let them take the lead it's remarkable what can occur. There were two or three major themes that came out, verbalized by the folks who were sitting at the front desk: the clerks, the radiology technicians, etc. Those themes ended up as key components of our next five-year strategic goal.

When I got here five years ago as corporate CEO, stretch goals or bonuses were already part of the compensation system, but nobody ever got paid anything. What I said to the board was, "Listen folks, I've got at least two years, maybe three years, to turn this situation around. Even though I may be under water for a couple of years, if I'm making improvement, I want to start getting some portion of these stretch goal bonuses out to people quickly. That's what will make them feel affirmed."

In the first year before we got above water, we started giving partial bonus payments. That was critical. I said, "If you don't want me to do this, it's up to you. You guys are the owners, but if you don't want me to do it, then let's get rid of this completely. It's even worse having it and not paying it."

After that first year, I can't tell you how many handwritten notes I got from people, saying, "My gosh, we've never experienced anything like this. Thank you so much." It's very concrete. We said to people that you are going to work harder, but you will really be happy because your own programs will be able to expand. You will be able to see the growth of your own programs. It's not just individual compensation; you will rebuild your residency programs, your specialty, and subspecialty care. You will have your community practice sites rebuilt, but only if we achieve these goals, both company goals as well as your individual work unit goals. It took a couple of years before there were groups that were actually experiencing that.

A bonus plan was designed, and it occurred to us that we ought to be doing something for the rest of the staff. We worked with HR to develop an incentive for the clinic based nursing and other staff to encourage them to sign up patients.

We've had good success over the last few years with the physician compensation plan as a way to change behavior. The key is that it mirrors what's important to the organization. It doesn't take a lot of money—using bonuses and withholds on patient satisfaction scores is an important message. The compensation plan is well structured and fits with the shared vision. This has promise for us.

I was always on the lookout for nationally known people to be potential board members for Geisinger. The President of the Commonwealth Fund and I resonated on a number of issues about healthcare reimbursement. I asked her to come visit us at Geisinger. We asked her if she would consider coming on the board, and she did. That all happened about 3½ years ago, and she is now as much of a national advertiser for Geisinger as anyone I've ever seen. It's helped our board tremendously because she's such an extraordinarily high-profile individual.

We meet with the department director and operations manager every month to discuss specific issues that are important to them. They develop the agenda. It's not just a matter of us having regular meetings with a group and laying out the issues. The personal interaction is important to us. It helps us get a great deal done.

We need to encourage more clinically oriented and patient-oriented research. We had a great opportunity for a partnership with Bucknell University. It really met our needs, and I think it met theirs. We wanted to organize joint research projects between their biomechanical engineering group and our orthopedic and basic-surgery groups. We have recruited very good clinicians who are focused intently on patient care. To be able to link them up with folks who spend all their time thinking about research is a good thing.

Because of a four-year emphasis on improving clinic service, 80% of 220 primary care physicians can see a patient within 24 hours. Specialists strive to see patients within seven days. We did a series of learning experiences, pilot projects, and tests, based on Don Berwick's ideas, to figure out how to do it. We got agreement with leadership for new standards on patient waiting time. Teams and resources, like electronic records, reinforce this. Expectations and measures were built into the compensation system on an individual and organization level. I'm proud of my colleagues—that we have made this effort and sustained it over three years.

Integrated Team Approach

There are times when we are not as successful as we'd like to be. At one point, our hospital patient-satisfaction scores tanked. Four leaders looked into each other's eyes, and each took responsibility for actions. We all share ownership for performance. There was no backing away. We were all accountable. That kind of behavior grows out of the values of the organization.

The corporate CEO has a Friday morning meeting involving 30 people. I presented the most recent patient satisfaction score to that group. Early in the agenda, he said patient satisfaction in one area was not satisfactory. This was serious business that I needed to focus on. The CEO pays attention and is a part of celebrating when we do well and is intent on holding people accountable when we do not meet Geisinger standards. In his experience as a practicing surgeon, he understood that his relationships with patients and referring physicians were critical to patient outcomes and success as a practice. He wants to be sure everyone in our organization understands that. I was thinking that the tenor of my presentation had to be consistent with his mood. I made it brief and serious. A pall came over the room. As the meeting ended, a number of people approached me and offered condolences. The CMO stopped me and said, "You are not in this alone. We know we can make it different. I will lend the weight of my position to make sure we are working on this." I went back to our team to talk about the best practices that we know influence the outcomes when we are at the top of our game.

We have work teams in adult ICU focused on the Save 100,000 Lives campaign. One of the senior people, along with nurses and physicians, pulled together seven or eight things about respirator care. They worked the process with data and got everybody on board. They took the rate of respirator-related pneumonia cases from 14 per 1,000 days to under 4 per 1,000 days. They have rallied as a multidisciplinary team and sustained results for a year and a half.

My unit functions with accountability on a daily basis. Nurses, secretaries, and physicians have an ability to flex. The schedule is never what happens that day. If someone needs to be seen, they are. At the end of the day, they are tired, but proud.

I work in surgery in dermatology, and it's a wonderful place to work. We have a great team of people. The one thing that we have is teamwork and collaboration. From a nursing standpoint, if we go to one of the doctors and express a concern about a patient or about their attitude, they seriously listen to us. They don't put us down like, "Well, you're the nurse, and I'm the doctor." They just treat us like we are a team. That's very important.

One of the earliest things I remember was when I was on-call one weekend. The physician director called me saying, "Hey, I'm in the hospital. Why don't I just see your patients for you." He is a spectacular guy, and that set the tone. It is "other centered," not "me centered."

Grand rounds are so effective. The director says, "What do you all think?" The nurses have more experience than I have. I'll ask the nurse. The nurses are able and willing to say, "Why don't you try this?" We work as a team and use information from everybody.

I wish you could see my day. I'm a part of several teams—weight management, psychiatry, family practice, and breast cancer clinic. I work with many partners, and there is mutual respect. I am needed. I know I need them and will learn from them. There are these wonderful moments, talking about patients—where everyone's input is valued.

Being stuck within a department or silo is not that important here. You've got a project, and you can go to anyone and describe what needs to be done and get something done.

There are a number of ways people evaluate their care. We focus on building an integrated team approach. The hospitalist works with nursing staff and residents. Skill development and process improvement are keys. We wanted to do better, so, we contacted our leaders. They are very receptive. They act like they appreciate your call when you ask them to do something. I needed their help and didn't have the answers myself. I wasn't certain we could make something happen in a reasonable time, and I was wrong.

We wanted to engage the staff in making the hospitalist program clearer to patients. We brought the hospitalists together with nursing team leaders. It was an open session discussing where we were and what we wanted to change. I wondered if they felt the need to change. They did. The group came up with specific ideas. They understood the patient's concerns about knowing who was caring for them. They suggested a pamphlet describing what a hospitalist is and does.

We have a group of physicians that are located in State College, in the center of the state about 80 miles west of our main campus. We've been looking to develop that market. Someone has been going up there several days a week to expand business. A resident has been trained who will join the practice full time. The responsibility to make that practice work is shared. Care has been taken not to put someone out there all alone without support or feeling the remainder of the group did not cover them. It's been successful building up the market for that group.

About two or three years ago, three of us started talking about what is the relationship between physician satisfaction and the risk of malpractice. A high point for me was discovering how to ask questions. We explored physician satisfaction and physician productivity. We had a statistician who could analyze data. It turns out that the more productive the physicians are the more satisfied the patients are. Patient confidence, trust, and follow-through on treatment also correlate. The results were exciting. The process of working with these colleagues is verification that we are on the right track with priorities.

Believing in People

From my perspective, development is one of the strengths of this organization. I have felt that when I wanted to go in a new direction or the organization wanted to go in a new organization, it put its money where its mouth is. For example, I was here five years, and we needed somebody to do this kind of surgery that I do called Mohs surgery. It's a way of removing skin cancers. We couldn't attract anybody. I said, "Well, my wife and I would be willing to leave for a year and do it."

They supported me. They not only helped me find a place, but they kept my salary going. They helped me with my house, over $100,000. I got a salary as a fellow, and they said, "We want you to maintain your standard of living while you are away. Then you just come back and get back to the organization." That was incredible.

So when we got involved in the service initiative, they put their money where their mouth was again. I told them that I needed to learn about service, so they sent me to Disney. They sent me to Mayo. They sent me all over. They said, "You tell me what you need to do to learn." So I looked at organizations, and I said, "This is where I need to go. This is where I need to study."

I was a big hitter at the time, meaning I made a lot of money for the organization. I went to them and said, "Listen, if I'm going to do this, I can't do that much surgery, and it's going to mean this many of hundreds of thousands of dollars reduction in productivity."

They said, "We think it's that important. We think you're the one to do it. You do it." It was unbelievable.

When I first came back from fellowship training in newborn intensive care, it was clear to me that our unit could be well served by a nurse practitioner program. I took a proposal for funding and got it. The program opened new worlds. A number of people were motivated to do more. When I explained what I wanted to accomplish, the medical director said, "I'm not sure I really understand the role or how it will change care, but I'm willing to take a chance. Just make it valuable, and maybe others can use the model."

I was really green. Only in retrospect did I realize how the willingness to take risk and trust is really important in moving the organization forward.

A high point was being asked in my second year of residency to stay on with a satellite clinic. I didn't know very much. The fact is this: They valued me enough to invite me to stay on. They saw potential and took a risk.

The types of recognition that mean the most are the unexpected—one- or two-line handwritten notes from colleagues that say, "Thanks for a great job on this." A former CEO sent me a set of little monographs that were the history of Geisinger Medical Center and a collection of historical papers from the first surgeon. As I opened them, there were personal notes from him. Those things are so memorable. They last.

I wish I had 30 more years because it's exciting, especially as we see what's happening with the technology. It's fun to learn, and we learn every day. I wish that the group of people that are here would continue in that vein and that the people who are hired will be people like them. I suspect that they will be because I think they attract similar people.

I would hope that this is the best dermatology department in the country. I mean it has the potential to be that because of the people who are here. The people are talented. They are good at what they do, and they are great people. If you put all that talent together and if they collaborate, they can create a department that is just superb.

Peak Experiences

Peak experiences occur frequently as a dermatologist. I find them when I have a patient that comes in and is fearful. I try to alleviate their anxiety. One patient left saying, "I just have to hug you." There is this emotional release. They thank me profusely when I call to follow-up. This morning I did surgery on a woman. When I called her later, she had just taken the dressing off her face, and she said, "Thank you. You were who I needed you to be." I helped her through the experience.

In December 2000, a team went to Jamaica on a medical outreach program. An American nun asked doctors to see a dying girl, age 15. She had a blistering skin disease in its worst form. She weighed 60 pounds and would have died within a week. Her skin, eyes, and esophagus were blistered. She couldn't swallow her own saliva or food. The doctors sent her, along with her mother, to Geisinger for treatment for two weeks. The girl said, "The director was right there when I came at midnight. He wanted to make sure I arrived safely."

The dermatology department took her on completely. She has a permanent tracheotomy, and is blind. Throughout treatment, she has never complained once. "Everyday I'd see the same doctor come in after hours, and that was the director." Two weeks turned into six years. The medical visa was repeatedly renewed for her and her mother. The director said, "She is my daughter. My family will walk the journey with her."

She started high school here at age 16 and graduated with honors after four years. She's a brilliant girl. She is 21 now and got a scholarship to Susquehanna U. The medical impact is significant. The world will be a better place because of her. She is going to make a difference in the world. This is a story of life coming from ashes.

While working in NICU, we are occasionally delaying the inevitable. A baby had a lung disease and was suffering. All of the ventilators in the world could not help. Some parents want to be there—others don't. This single mom did not feel she could be there for the baby's demise. I was the physician responsible and said to one of the nurses, "This is just awful. This little guy is going to live his entire life inside the confines of the ICU."

We took the baby off the ventilator. I got security to unlock the doors and went upstairs to the outside play deck. It was a nice October evening, with a beautiful sunset. The nurse checked back with me after calling the mother to let her know what was happening. I was holding the baby while in a swing that looked to the east at a bank of trees that were orange and yellow. The last time we heard the heartbeat was as the shadows came off the pine trees. The baby died in my arms.

I tell this story to new residents to encourage them to share what they are involved in with their families. There are so many things that raise questions that we don't have answers for and that have meaning we don't understand. That's part of the wonder of the practice of medicine.

There's a camp in Minnesota for kids sponsored by the Academy of Dermatology. We thought, "We should do a camp. We can do a skin camp." It took a lot of collaboration because we had no money. We sold pins and called drug companies. We celebrated our 10th year last year.

In the beginning, we took mainly local kids so that we didn't have to pay for planes. The first year we took 30 kids for four days. We now have 90 kids, mostly from the United States and a few from other countries—New Zealand, Bermuda, and Canada. There are ten of us who go down on three buses to Harrisburg, Pennsylvania. Occasionally, with that many kids, 60 or so on planes, we have to stay over. Once I was in a motel with five or six kids and only two beds. Of course, nobody wants to sleep with someone else. We took the mattresses apart. I slept on the springs. Once they are there, the camp is a seamless operation. There are well over 50 people working there—residents, practicing physicians, and other volunteers. We have a Med Shed where we have a staff of nurses. We have a volunteer doctor from Akron, Ohio who helps with the fishing. There are activities coordinated from morning till night. It gives these kids, many of whom are blistered from head to toe with bandages, a chance to go right in the swimming pool. The bandages come off. It's been the only opportunity for so many with no hands and no fingers. It is just something so good. The highlight for me is watching the joy on the kids' faces because they are not concerned about how they look. The other kids look the same with bandages and blisters. They can be who they are. Once we had motorcyclists that came out and gave them rides, bandanas and all. One little guy said, "I just held on to his tummy, and it was real squishy."

I was interested in how we might develop a measure of clinical outcomes in rheumatic disease. I sat down with a doctor who knows a great deal about technology and databases. I laid out an idea and asked him to work on it. He developed a database that is still in use in rheumatology. What came out of that was a relationship that has been important to both of us over the years.

I had always wondered why, in a certain inflammatory disease, people were weak. No one had really looked at and understood it. I went to my colleague and said, "Have you ever given any thought to why people are weak in this disorder?" I simply posed the question. He took the idea and developed it into a research project, and it launched his interest in clinical research. He took the idea far beyond my wildest dreams and is now nationally known. It's been a very nice evolving relationship. We rely on each other for guidance and direction.

I went to a dermatology conference recently. There was a session done by an older physician from Mayo on work–life balance. My wife said, "You need to go to it." I asked him a question about the constant issue of adding patients and feeling overwhelmed. He said, "If I add patients to the point where I am not truly listening and caring about what they are saying, then I've added too many." That answered the question about "what's too much."

Yesterday I had an experience that reinforced that. A fellow I had seen many years ago came in and told me his wife died. He got teary. I realized he needed time to be heard. I asked him to tell me about it. He said, "God is helping me through it. Living alone is hell. I hate it." When he left, he said, "Can I give you a hug? I love you, doctor." The reason he said that is because I listened to him. That was a powerful lesson. I'll never forget that one. It was a fabulous experience.

I had one gentleman that had been seen by various dermatologists. He was head to toe just pure blood. He was dripping in the room with blood on his clothes. He said, "I have become an expert of washing blood out of clothes. This is what I look like."

I said to him, "We are going to have to do something a lot higher risk than you've been doing before—something systemic that suppresses your immune system to get you some relief. You can't live like this anymore."

We talked about a couple of different medications, the side effects, and all of the risks. He was a little bit hesitant, and I was a little bit hesitant; however, we decided to try one. We did blood tests and checked everything out and then got him started on it. In a month or two, we slowly increased the dose and watched his blood tests. He cleared—no more blood. He looked like a new man. He did so incredibly well. Every time I see him now he gives me this big hug. Last time I called him with his blood test results to say, "Hey, everything is okay. Everything is looking good. How have you been?"

He said, "You know—they are going to change the name of the hospital to name it after you."

I said, "What?"

He said, "Well after they get my patient satisfaction form, they are going to want to change the name of that hospital." That was, of course, very, very rewarding. It is always enjoyable to have that kind of relationship develop with patients. I'm starting to learn that the more time that goes along—how much of a relationship you can develop with these patients.

In 1995, I had a visit from one of the vice presidents, and that's not good. Whenever vice presidents visit you it's been my experience that either you're in trouble or they want something. They don't usually come down to pat you on the back and say, "Great job. Great to see you. Just thought I'd wander by."

We talked pleasantries, and finally, he said, "We are going to embark on a new initiative. We are refocusing this organization around better service. We are going hold a retreat of all of the heads of the departments and administrative counterparts."

I was thinking, "I'm not the head of a department. Why is he telling me?"

He said, "We would like you to come. I would like you to present this to the medical staff. You provide great service."

So I went to this retreat. I can't remember what I said to the medical staff, but what was fascinating was their reaction. I got e-mails and people stopping me in the hall saying, "It's about time. Thanks for talking about this." It was incredible.

About six months later, I got a call from the CEO. He said, "I want you to come to the System Planning Retreat with all of the big people in the whole system. We strategize and develop tactics. I want you to give us an update on where we are with service."

I said, "We are nowhere. We haven't done a thing. I gave an address to the medical staff and that was it."

"I want you to come and give us an update anyway." So I went and I challenged them. I read these three questions:

"Is service excellence a worthy goal? Do we have the will and energy to pursue it? And can we agree on a plan and implement?"

The CEO stood up and said, " He's right. We are in the service business. I will commit this organization to developing a plan and implementing it. Does anybody have any questions?"

I am sitting back there thinking, "Don't ask any questions." This neurosurgeon, a crusty old guy, raised his hand and said, "Yeah, I have a question. What do you mean by service excellence? Give me an example."

I blurted out real quickly, "I don't know, like serving coffee and cookies in the waiting room." This guy went like this (shrug). Here I was a dermatologist, who he probably thinks I squeeze pimples all day, telling him you need to serve tea and crumpets in the waiting room. He thought I'd gone mad.

What I realized at that point was I didn't know what I was talking about. I knew it was right, but I didn't know how to teach it. From that point on, I went back to my desk and learned about service. Not only what exceptional service means, but how to go to your department and implement it.

I got the organizational leadership to commit to measuring, with a significant investment of money. The point made was that if we're going to do it, we are going to do it right. I am not going to screw around with this. I've got a nice clinic. It's fun, and I'm not going to do this half baked. So if you want to do this, put the money up and commit to measuring it, and take the measurement tool to drive process improvement. Let's measure it by physician! That was something that was tough to convince them of.

We got leadership to buy off. You probably heard we've made some pretty significant strides. In retrospect, it was something I'm really proud of. This organization is still working on it. That was the genesis.

Developing Others

There are three types of events that always go well in developing people at Geisinger. We do a half-day orientation on service excellence for new people. It gets positive feedback. They see quickly that healthcare is a lot deeper than the tasks involved, and they understand why striving for excellent service really matters.

Then we do individual coaching sessions for people who have low scores in patient satisfaction. After they get past the initial resistance, they end up feeling that they benefit from it. Finally, we offer workshops on improving service using hands-on observing and practicing. We hire a local acting group to play patients.

You know, if you are an athlete, you watch films all week long. If you are in a theater production, you have producers watching you and taking notes. You watch other actors and actresses. In almost every other field, you watch other people, and you see how they work. Physicians don't. They will talk about disease process, diagnosis, treatment, and medicine, but they are alone in making a connection with a patient. So I have no idea that my colleague right beside me is able to make a fantastic connection in a difficult situation. I never get to see the colleague do it. We figured out how to do this. Working in small groups with typical patients allows physicians to watch each other interact with patients.

Physicians practice alone. They don't automatically make connections with patients. One of the best things we do is a workshop with actors. We ask the physicians, "What kind of things are you struggling with?" They give an example.

The actor plays the patient. We talk about how to help the situation. The doctors gain insight in how to make a connection with a patient. We bring into practice things that other doctors have found that work. After a workshop, one doctor came to me and said, "I tried it and it worked. I could see the relief come over the patient."

We try to drive home the idea, Isn't it odd that in the medical profession, more than others, we don't coach each other? Coaching with actors is one way of getting us to do that. Even though there's a focus on trying to teach patient relations in school, there is so much science and content to learn. The relationship I have with my patients is more important than the facts. People like the director and his team role model getting the relationship right so well that we look to him and his team for how it comes together

I was at a workshop one or two years ago with a new colleague. We talked about improving the residency program. Three of us who were interested went to her and said, "What can we do to improve communication skills of residents?" Together, we created a wonderful program, with education and sophisticated evaluation to address salient problems.

We design classes and experiences that make their practice better. It's a creative process. We tell stories. We use actors as patients. We design educational experiences to take concepts into practice.

The corporate CEO asked me to design a physician leadership program for clinicians with potential from inside Geisinger. He was surprised folks weren't percolating to the top. I drew on my own experience and looked at the people who are clinical leaders. What set of competencies did they exhibit? We provided experiences where they would see senior leaders in action and see parts of the organization they wouldn't normally see. The program is in the CMO's budget, which demonstrates that it's a priority for the organization. We created a brochure to explain the program and use as a personal invitation. We now have six physicians a year in the program. We want the best place for physician leaders to be right here.

Coaching and Being Coached

Residents come in every July. They see a patient and present the patient to us. Countless times, the resident will say to me. "I have a lady in this room, a 56-year-old lady."

I say, "What's her name?"

"I don't know."

"Really. Well, we have to know her name. You've got to know who the person is to have a relationship."

Initially, it just doesn't hit them that you really have to create a relationship in everything you do. That's what you want. You can develop a relationship, you and I, in a couple of minutes, as though we've known each other. We can be friends and pick up right where we left off. Whereas if you refer to somebody as "oh, that lady I saw yesterday with. . . ." Who was it? The woman has a life-threatening disorder, and she's "that lady." Who is it?

It happened to me in an emergency room one time when somebody said, "Who's in bed 8?" The reply was, "It's that lady dying from congestive failure." I thought, "That lady dying?" It's her last moments, and she doesn't have a name? It's scary.

This is part of our service standards. "What's the person's name?" If you don't know how to pronounce the name, ask them. Then you call him by that name.

This is a very natural way to teach the importance of names. I can do this without really thinking about it. I just do it naturally because I have been doing it for a long time. What we see with residents after they are here for a few months is that they are doing it. They are all doing it, and they do have relationships with people. It makes their work more fun or more meaningful because they are seeing people as human beings—not just as a disease.

One person has been a role model for me. I stay close to him. He asks, "Do you want to write part of this article? Do you want to speak?" He helps me achieve in academics. That first year I saw him teaching residents in a way I've never experienced. During my fellowship, I took this with me. I pulled residents aside, and we showed slides every week. When I came back, I took over the role of teaching. I emulate his teaching.

About three years ago, we were looking at our programs in physician communication and service delivery. We needed to broaden our expertise, specifically with physicians who have difficulty. Our psychologist came to work in our department, part time. His focus is on doctors who score low on patient satisfaction surveys and are having challenges getting along on teams. We suspected he had tremendous potential. I had no clue how to do this. I hoped he knew what to do. It was clear in looking at his face that he was enthused. The gears were churning in his head. He said yes before he left the room. He came back with an outline. It was really good work. I said, "I'm so glad we asked you to think about this because it can really take us forward."

Coaching was a void in our training. We were not ever explicitly trained to be coaches. It was not part of medical school. I really think to learn to coach others in a way that actually helps the other person is not enough of a focus. We are fortunate to have just hired someone in education, with expertise in curriculum development and helping medical residents be better teachers. They learn how to coach and provide feedback as a continuous process. That is unique here. We are helping residents become teachers beyond their specialty knowledge. Teaching staff, patients, and other doctors is part of their role.

Loyalty to the Patient

Patients have the doctor's e-mail addresses and their home phone. They have everything.

I went downstairs one day to wait for a food delivery person. This little old lady who might have been 80 years old came up to me as I was standing there and said, "Does this bus go to Shamokin?"
    I said, "The shuttle bus?"

"Yeah, I need to get home, and I don't know how to get home."

"This bus only goes to our parking lot, ma'am."

She said, "Well, I need to get home. I don't know how to get home."

I said, "How did you get here?"

"I was brought in by ambulance last night in the ER. I'm tired. I'm hungry. I haven't had anything to eat."

Now, I am waiting for a big food delivery to arrive. So I said, "Do you have anyone—a neighbor or someone—who can come get you? Anyone?"

"No, I don't know any of my neighbors."

There's this poor little soul out in the middle of nowhere, and she just didn't know where to go. She wasn't a dermatology patient, but we contacted Social Services. Geisinger bought her a ticket for a taxi to get back home again. I got her food. Our department isn't generous to only the dermatology patients. We will go above and beyond for whatever patients there are—wherever and whatever their needs are. I think it's a great place to work. I anticipate working there for the rest of my life, the next 25 years.

I've been with Geisinger for 17 years. I started out on the Med–Surg floor where we did a lot of wound care. We never got to actually see the patient being healed, where in dermatology we see these patients every week. We develop a rapport, and they become like your family. It's so great just seeing them heal. It's a long process, and you get to watch them and see them heal. You get to see them smile and say thank you.

So many times we get patients that come in, and they will say they saw a doctor at another hospital who "wants to cut my leg off." Our physician director has saved so many limbs. He does not give up hope. I can count at least a dozen patients where he's actually saved their limbs. They say, "I might lose my leg in a year or two, but I will never look back and say, 'What if we tried this? What if I did this?'" They know that everything was done that was possible for them.

When you talk about dermatology, they hire for success. It's very important for them to have people who are qualified. Candidates have to demonstrate clearly that they are going to commit to the values and show it in their behavior at work. It's difficult to change people's fundamental values if they are not committed to patient service and that relationship—the real interest in the patient. They are not going to fit with patient's expectations, and they won't fit with those around them. "I do my job—they got their appointment." That's not going to work in dermatology. They won't understand why those around them are frustrated. It's not fair to hire them. The dermatology department has been very diligent in their hiring and looking at the total picture—in looking at what a resident, staff person, nurse, or receptionist will bring to the table.

Service Hero Stories

Our leaders know the value of the stories to inspire but need to know that it is also a strategy for change leadership.

We collect stories from in-house, and once every six months we select service heroes. A ceremony takes place in the medical center auditorium. I will usually tell one or two stories, and we'll have six people lined up to tell stories. What an uplifting event this is! I get e-mails and calls from people. You can see how the room is engaged. We talk about the differences we make. You see family members feeling being proud and leaders feeling proud. There are things that go on here every day that are nothing less than heroic. I'll tell people that at 9/11 we discovered who our heroes were. We thought heroes were athletes and movie stars. Our heroes are everyday people who go out of their way when they are called on to make a difference. Stories are a reward for the service heroes and a chance for people to share, grow, and learn from the stories.

We believe that these stories are valuable enough in helping our own culture that we created a program to pull them out. Thus, we collect stories of our own that we will tell in different forums. This is something that goes very, very well. For example, one of those stories involves a radiology tech and a 9-year-old girl who got hysterical because of sedation for an MRI. They pulled out the big long needle, and she freaked. The family freaked, and they couldn't get her calmed down. The next alternative was general anesthesia to just knock her out. There are a lot of reasons why you don't want to do that.

One of our techs came over to her and said, "Honey, what do you think if you and I did this together? Do you think you can do it if I did it with you?" And the little girl thought that maybe she could. So they held hands, and rolled up the sleeves, and we started the needle in the tech's arm and the 9-year-old's arm.

Now, we don't have any job descriptions that say you have to get stuck with needles. I always enjoy telling this story, and I say, "Don't worry. We didn't sedate our employees. We are not drugging our people." The bottom line is that somebody was thinking on their feet about what he or she could do in that moment to help this kid get through it.

I could spend the rest of the morning telling stories like that. In these forums, there's a mixture of our people, management, and senior management. When we celebrate we ask them to bring their families in as well. It's kind of neat that the families come. I get to tell the story in a very large room, and you can pretty much see the entire room just feeling good.

One of the reasons I look forward to service heroes is that I've found that people want and need to be inspired. As managers in health care, usually very little is done for us on the inspirational side. We manage reports, data, schedules, and issues. I am surprised how seldom people are told that they are doing meaningful and worthwhile work and that they are making a difference.

Storytelling has become part of our organization over the last decade. When you take a concept and translate it into a story, it shows what it means. We are much more into that. In an organization that continues to grow, with thousands of employees, when someone in a significant position of responsibility tells a personal story, it brings us all together and says, "What one person does among thousands is what we are all about." There were 1.5 million clinic visits last year. If I did 2,000 of them, what difference does that make? You understand that every time you are seeing a patient, you are making a difference.

Work Family

Back in 2002, I had a daughter who was very ill. She too is a Geisinger employee. She missed six months of work. Out of those six months, because of the generosity of my department, she only went without three weeks of pay. My department stood up and said that they were going to take care of this by donating their leisure time. How can you even begin to thank folks for that? That just goes to show you what a remarkable department this is. It's not a department. It's a family. Our team is our family. There is no discrepancy between staff, resident, secretary, receptionist, or whoever we are. We all work together. We are all there for the good of the patient. This will be my last job, but I will say that I have always been blessed to be a part of the hospital.

One of the things I see historically in dermatology is a work unit that accepts new people and gathers them into the group not only professionally but also socially. This includes the family. They have a much higher retention rate than those units who tell new hires, "Here is your office down the hall and here is your schedule, and we'll let you know if there is any problem."

Four years ago I got laid off after 32 years with Geisinger. I was hurt and angry. After four months, the people in dermatology let me know there was an opening. I was crying in the interview. They made me feel really welcome. They would only hire someone who fit. I felt like the best thing that happened to them. I want to retire here.

When I was part of the family practice residency, my father died about six years ago. Residents were a lot younger than I was. The residents were sympathetic and made sure that they said something about it. I hadn't realized that they were keeping track of my personal life. It turns out that they were. This is common here. There are sometimes very moving memorial experiences. At a memorial service for a colleague in pediatrics who died, one of our physician leaders said, "Life is about taking risks. . . . There are chances we take." He walked over to the piano and played for everyone.

What makes it pleasant for me is having things phrased as a request rather than a command. When you ask someone to do something, they will ultimately come back with a completed project. They may ask clarifying questions, but they proceed.

The patients here are great. They are appreciative, kind, and compliant. It's my home. It's fun to come to work. Today three people asked me if my grandfather was the one who ran the store. That happens to me every day. We have a clothing store downtown, and every time I think about leaving I think how everybody asks me about my granddad or my dad being a lawyer in town. So those things are fun.

We had a patient who went shopping and bought us all a ceramic Christmas ornament. We collected money, bought a tree, and sent her a picture of the decorated tree.

One of the things I liked about Geisinger is the professional, yet informal, relationship among staff. Physicians make jokes with nurses. We are at ease with each other.

I will never leave this department. Everyone treats you with kindness and respect. The nurses and doctors work harder than we do.

I wouldn't want to leave here because I already enjoy it now. Why would I want to go anywhere else? It's just a great place to work.

Editor Commentary

The leadership at Geisinger, particularly the physician leaders, has embraced a philosophy of "both/and"—technical quality and service quality as being equally essential to individual patient outcomes and the success of the entire organization.

It seems like everyone understands this "both/and"—patients want and need their technical skills—but they are equally focused on being extraordinary communicators. This manifests itself in staff members having a special antenna for identifying and responding to patients' feelings, and all staff members are comfortable suggesting to each other how best to meet a patient's particular needs. Compassion shows through big and small examples; the statement "the patients live in their world not ours" speaks volumes.

Staff members—physicians, clinicians, and nonclinical employees—express a tremendous amount of pride (but not a hint of arrogance) in the work that they do and the overall level of quality care that Geisinger delivers. Staff members at all levels share a sense of humility and talk of being honored to have the opportunity to serve patients and family members as part of a team of incredibly talented and dedicated professionals. Staff members at all levels mentioned their sense of inclusion—whether at organization-wide visioning sessions or informal "what do you think?" meetings. A high degree of collegiality and mutual respect is apparent at all staff levels.

Education—both of new physicians and ongoing learning by all staff members—plays an essential role in the Geisinger story. There are numerous references to teaching (and learning)—by role modeling, first and foremost. Humbleness permeates the organization, which spurs additional discovery—we know a lot, but we don't everything (whether this is about how to treat a patient or how to organize a journey to service excellence)—and creates a platform for increased personal, professional, and organizational growth.

The organization values risk taking as well and actively engages in supporting those who are "trying something new." In particular, the bold statement of giving "partial bonuses or not at all" stands as a defining moment in their already decade-old and still-continuing journey. Risk taking is apparent in many more subtle ways, such as the acknowledgment that much of what makes Geisinger physicians special isn't taught in medical school. This is a radical and risky admission for most physicians to make—and yet has driven many of the most inspirational improvements—in coaching, education, and patient care at this organization.

Table 8-1 Organizational Demographics

Organization	Mountain States Health Alliance
Location	Johnson City, TN
Setting	Suburban
Communities served	Suburban and rural
Type of organization	Private, not for profit community and academic medical center
Number of beds	1,199
Number of FTEs	5,800
Scope of service	JCMC is a community-based, academic medical center hosting residents, medical students, and public and allied health students from East Tennessee State University. JCMC is a level I trauma center with the region's most active open heart and comprehensive cardiac program, the Regional Cancer Center, the St. Jude's Clinic, the Center for Women's Health, the Children's Hospital, a regional renal and pancreatic transplant program, and a full range of medical and surgical specialties. MSHA owns 11 hospitals and over 20 medical practices.
Organizational awards	Magnet Recognition, Top 100 Heart Hospital, Excellence Award for the Tennessee Center for Performance Excellence, Most Wired Hospital, Blue Cross Blue Shield Distinction for Cardiac Services, two MSHA facilities winner of Compass Awards for patient satisfaction, CARF accreditation
Focus area	Johnson City Medical Center
	Joint Replacement Center
Focus area	MSHA President's Award for Quality
Best practices and awards	TVC recognition
	Current patient satisfaction above the 90th percentile

The Power of Storytelling

Contributors: Carolyn Rainey Weisenberger and Cheri B. Torres

The stories in this chapter are the voices of the senior executive team for Mountain States Health Alliance, the CEO and CNO of Johnson City Medical Center, the senior director for guest services, two patient care directors, nurse managers, nurses, patient care staff, physicians, patients, and members of the community. Here are their stories.

MOUNTAIN STATES HEALTH ALLIANCE

The Power of Storytelling

Approximately four years ago, the team at Mountain States decided that we were going to embark on a journey to bring love and care to healthcare. Part of that was celebrating the patients as individuals and recognizing that patients have individual needs and have individuality that they bring to the healthcare setting. So we began celebrating religious preferences and their personal preferences by talking and listening more to our patients. It quickly became evident that oftentimes stories are a vehicle in which we communicate with one another, a way in which we share some of those ideals. Shortly after that, the International Storytelling Center and our Mountain States Foundation came together and decided to help us with the application of storytelling inside the facility. Our initial intent was to provide diversion to patients.

The International Storytelling Center is located six miles from our main facility, and each year professional storytellers from all over the world come to celebrate the craft of storytelling. They let us come down to their facility and tape those professional storytellers. We began to play those inside the health-care facility on the in-house network. It became quickly evident that those stories provided certainly diversion, but they also provided stories of hope. People tend to connect with other folks' stories; so, they would see themselves in another story, and they would find comfort, hope, or diversion in the stories. It took off quickly in terms of our patients and our family members enjoying the application of storytelling.

Our mission is to bring love and care to health care. If we truly want to achieve this, then we need to listen to our patients and meet them where they are in their journey and in their story. As we attempt to find out more about the patient or the family and their expectations for their healthcare experience or try to set expectations for their healthcare experience, oftentimes stories are great vehicles to frame both of those things. Our mission is to create an environment that will heal the mind, body, and spirit. Certainly storytelling touches the mind and the spirit, and it captures the essence of people caring for people.

Patients have their own unique belief system and identity. Oftentimes those identities come out in conversations that we have or those stories that we tell. Every person that is a patient in a hospital certainly was a person before they came to us. We need to listen to their stories to help us frame them as a person and give them an identity. We also need to share stories with them that perhaps might help them as they complete the healing process.

For instance, in the Joint Replacement Center, we use the application of stories in a unique way. A great story of inspiration is to think about what you will be doing once you have your joint replaced. Patients share those stories frequently about "when I get out of this hospital I'm going to climb that mountain" or "I'm going to go on that hike" or "I'm going to go on that ski slope" or "I'm going to get out on that tractor." All of those give patients identities, and they are their stories.

We implemented a Mountain States Mission Moment, which is a five- to seven-minute communication time that occurs twice each day throughout our facility. We designed it to share information about operations, a new policy, a new form, a new procedure, but also, it's a way that we can celebrate the successes that occur within Mountain States. So oftentimes that five-minute moment may contain a patient story. It may be that a patient sent us a letter with his or her story about what being in the hospital meant. When you do that you connect the dots for the caregiver who's on the floor. They are part of that wonderful patient experience. So, it not only is good for the patient, but for the team members as well. It creates that sense of purpose, and that sense of purpose is bringing love and care to health care.

We have a number of interviewing techniques that are used inside Mountain States. We offer educational programs that deal with patient–doctor or patient–staff interactions. The use of storytelling might be nothing more than "let's talk about how we take a history and physical." We also have another program called the VIP Program (Very Important Partner) in which a patient can designate a family member to be more intricately linked to their health-care information. We communicate frequently with that partner as well so that it gives us another connection to that healthcare team. We have a form called the Healing Tree that we place in our patient rooms. It provides an opportunity for us to mark down those things that are important to patients—whether it's people in their lives or activities they enjoy. It gives us a springboard for which to start those conversations with patients. Then the focus becomes what's important to the patient, not necessarily what's important to that transaction of health care.

I'll tell you a story. We had a patient in our ICU several months ago. Her Healing Tree noted the importance of music to her. So we started bringing music into her room. We had a harpist who would come in and play for her, and actually, on the day she died, our harpist was present. We will never know from that patient's perspective the impact that had, but we had to think from a patient who had a love for music we were able to create an environment for her that was very specific to that patient. So her story was not manifested in words, but it was manifested in the information that we got from the Healing Tree.

The mayor of one of our local communities was in the hospital, and she didn't know about Stories for the Soul: the storytelling channel. She said that she turned the television on and was channel surfing and serendipitously came upon Stories for the Soul. She said, "It was amazing to me how quickly my focus changed from, 'Oh, my gosh, I'm sick, I'm in the hospital, I don't feel good' to being taken away to different places through those stories." So when she recounts her experience of Stories for the Soul, she said it immediately reminded her that there is life outside this hospital, and it really truly was heal-ing. She said, "I could listen to those stories and think, 'Wait a minute when I get out of here I want to go back to the Storytelling Center' or 'I want to go back down to my grandmother's house.'" Listening to those stories really cele-brated life for her and allowed her think of her own story.

I used creative storytelling to help merge two of the hospital systems when we first formed the alliance. One of the hospitals we acquired was an alcohol and drug rehabilitation hospital. Another one of our facilities had one floor that was devoted to this same type of healthcare service. The logical move was to merge the staff from both hospitals. This, of course, meant all of the potential challenges that arise when uniting two different ways of doing business. I sent out wedding invitations to the hospital folk that would be involved. Our hospital chaplain was the lucky person to perform the mock wedding for the "family and friends" of the "bride and groom," and then we all celebrated at a reception party. This was one of the most powerful moments we experienced in our transition. What could have been a disaster full of conflict turned into something really positive.

I started the Monday Morning Newsletter really before I ever came to Mountain States as the CEO. I started it at my previous job. I tried to find a good way to communicate with people in the hospital; so, I put out a newsletter, and I just kept it going. I've been doing it for about 10 years. Sharing my stories and the stories of others is a way to develop the culture in the organization. I try to write something that is going to touch somebody, build morale in some way, and make people think. I send this out to all of the physicians on the staff and the community leaders. Many of the community leaders take it and use it in their workplace.

It all began with an elevator ride when I said good morning to a gentleman. He looked up and said, "Well?"

When I asked, "Is it only a morning today? Not really good yet?"

He replied, "Well, no." Then he looked at my hair and said, "You know, in WW II, they said blonds have more fun." I told him I thought it was funny that he thought I was a real blond. Then I thought, "I think there's a story there." So I asked, "What service were you in?"

"Well, I was in the Navy, Army, and Air Force." Now this was like from the sixth floor to the first floor. When we got off the elevator, he was still talking, and so, I went around the corner with him. I told him he'd been through a lot and that I bet the tests that we are going to put him through today probably are not as rough as what he'd already been through.

He kind of looked and said, "You know—you may be right." He smiled and started down the hall. I thought that was a brief encounter, but hopefully his telling that story helped him to get through something. It was quite a neat experience.

Connecting With Patients

I couldn't believe the afternoon of the day I was operated on the nurse came in and said, "Let's get you up. We're going to Roane Mountain."

"Roane Mountain?" I said. "I just had surgery!" She said, "I know. We gotta get you up and moving even if we only walk to Bull's Gap!"

They have all of the area's mountains painted on the walls, and each one represents a different walking distance. They do get you up and moving right away, though. With my nurse's encouragement and loving care, I walked just a bit that first day despite the pain, and by the next day, I walked to Roane Mountain—down the hall!

I'd have another joint replaced today if I needed it. The care I received was incredible. There were no surprises, and the staff was wonderful. Whatever you wanted you got!

This is like family for us; we'll do anything for each other as well as for the patients and doctors. Even the administrative staff will do things for patients when it's not their job. Like the other day when a patient needed water and we were all busy with other things, the secretary responded to the call light and filled a patient's water pitcher, and I've seen our housekeeper sense that a patient wanted company stop to visit with her for a while.

Our night nurse, Nikki, is just incredible. She loves to make crafts, and for every holiday and season, she'll create things for each patient's door, for our desks, and sometimes for every team member. She and her family sometimes wear costumes and visit with patients on special holidays. She's created a great photo board in the staff room to remind us of all of the fun we have!

I have conversations with my managers all of the time, "Thanks for doing this. This is a great thing." One manager saw a patient in need who didn't have any resources and didn't have money. She was concerned about her appearance. He arranged to take her down, paid for a hairdo in a salon, and sent her a bouquet of flowers. He did something specifically for a patient that really made her stay better.

I want everybody to be treated exactly as if it was your mother, your father, your sister, your brother, or your child. I don't care who they are, what color skin they have, whether they're rich or poor, whether they are a board member, or whether they live under the bridge. Everybody needs to be treated alike. I give the example of my father who was an alcoholic, and it might be my father that shows up in the emergency room. He might be drunk. He might be acting out, but he's somebody's dad. We need to think about that when we are taking care of these people and make sure that they are treated with love and respect. He might not be in his right mind at that particular time, but we've got to show him the love as if he were our own family member who is going through this crisis in his life.

I was dreading the day because I had worked probably 60 plus hours that week, but I knew that we needed help because the census was high. Truly I did not want to come in because I was just frazzled, but once I got here, I had this inner peace. I recognized that I was doing something good that day. I tell my patients all of the time if I can make a difference in one person's life today I've done my job, and that's what keeps me coming back.

As manager, I had come in to do an extra shift to help out on the unit. I was displaced, and I wasn't working somewhere that I normally work. I had a patient who was obviously very depressed, very distraught. You could just really tell it in her eyes that she was just having a lot of stress. It was a busy day, and I noted it on my assessment that morning. I knew I wanted to go back to see her when I looked in her eyes that morning. She just had this distant look in her eyes. It was almost eerie. I could tell by her mannerisms and her body language that something was wrong. She was very guarded, with her covers pulled up, and I know that she wanted to touch. I was trying to fix her covers, and she would touch and would look up. She was almost to the point that she wanted to cry. I could just tell that she needed something more than my other patients.

I just had five patients that day, which is a typical day. The acuity was not high at all, but I knew she was going to take some time because she had had extensive procedures. She had multiple dressings, and she was a very heavy lady, probably 400 plus pounds; so, she was sort of at my mercy because she couldn't move. She couldn't roll. So I got some free time later that day and went in there and talked to her. She told me that this was a newly diagnosed thing. She had had renal cancer, and it had eaten into the bone, into her hips. She had had a hip caging and all this extensive instrumentation, and it had become infected. She said until about four months prior she was carrying on a full-time job, the family, the whole gamut of things, and this had just really paralyzed her. She was facing a revision of all this extensive work secondary to her cancer. So she did not want to go on with life. She was just at the end of her rope. They were going to send her to Vanderbilt for this surgery because we couldn't provide that level of care here.

So I intervened and said, "What can we do here to keep her here because she was going to be traveling and would be in the hospital for several months?" This was a major stressor. Her family couldn't come, and she was going to be by herself. She had a life-changing event happen, and I don't know about her support group because I looked around and there was nobody there. After speaking with her, I did find out that she had a husband at home and that he was somewhat supportive, but he was having issues with her not being able to work. I knew that she needed something extra, and I was going to do whatever it took.

So we involved case management, and I had the clergy come from the hospital come up and talk to her. Long story short, we got everybody involved, and I got someone to assume her case here. I included the orthopedic doctors, case management, social work, and everybody involved. I even had the family come in and help make some of the decisions.

That was the first time in 10 years that a patient has ever made me cry, and I think that's what makes this stand out. She is back in on my unit now, doing well. She is actually just back in for antibiotic treatment. We got all of the hardware and infection removed from her body, and she's progressing well. They thought that she was going to be terminal, and it turned out that it wasn't so. I went in and talked to her just the other day, and she said, "You made such a difference in my life." She said, "I don't know if you realize that or not, but I think God sent you that day because I needed you." We have formed a really terrific bond, she and I. We have that professional relationship, but we also have a very special friendship that has come out of it. I think that's probably something that's made me proud because that's what I do every day. I probably do take it for granted, but I know that I'm in the right profession. It's really and truly a calling, and I think things happen and God puts you places you need to be for those people who need you.

Patients Supporting Each Other

Mountain State Health Alliance's Joint Replacement Center is cutting edge. It was designed from the ground up to serve the patient's best healthcare interests. They schedule surgery in groups. All knees come into the hospital on the same day and leave at the same time and all shoulders, etc.; so we got to know each other well and encouraged one another.

We all attended an introductory session together before we came for surgery. We learned about everything that was going to happen to us, and we got a book that gave us all the details. We couldn't have wanted any more information, including what to do afterward and what exercises to do to continue our rehab work on our own. We had our physical therapy on the floor together and shared a picnic lunch together just before we left. So we got to know one another. We really kind of felt like we were all in this together.

Then we all got together at the annual reunion. That was fun—it felt sort of like a family reunion. People with all kinds of joint replacements came.

We all brought photos of ourselves doing things we couldn't do before surgery. I saw some great shots of guys fishing and golfing again and older ladies playing golf or doing yoga.

One thing that we did with our joint center was to have a reunion with our patients. We tried to plot the course of where we wanted to go, which is that we want to improve outcomes with our patients. Through those efforts, we were able, like a year later, to have a reunion of our patients. I think when we brought all of those patients together we were able to demonstrate what we were about and what we had tried to accomplish. It was exciting and fun. We had a team of our folks who went up and decorated the room. We tried to make it pleasant. We had good food, and we wanted to make it a fun day. As a spinoff from that day, we also offered patients the opportunity to be ambassadors for our program. From that group, we have about 13 of our previous patients who now serve as our ambassadors. They will do some of our PR things, and then they will also, if we have patients with questions about the program, serve as a resource for them.

When you go to our unit, you will see that we have patients' pictures on the wall. We've got one man who is riding his horse and one who is plowing the garden. We have pictures of people with their dogs and with their grandchildren. We can see that we've made an impact on patients' lives in a positive way, and it's kind of a reaffirmation to see the pictures the wall.

Patients First

We are protective of our patients and families. I remember one situation that made me famous throughout the organization. One of our hospital executives had back surgery. He was very well known and loved throughout the organization. We had an issue with visitation: Everybody wanted to see him. We had to kind of cull that because it wasn't really helping him. He needed time to rest and recuperate.

He would not put his brace on unless I was there. He wouldn't get up unless I was there. He became very dependent on me because of the relationship that was established with him as a patient. He had never been on "that side of the bed" before.

One day we had done several things, and he was really tired. He told me he needed to rest some. I said, "No problem."

When I was out at the desk the CEO came in and I said, "May I help you, Sir?"

He said, "I'm going to see your patient."

I said, "No, he's actually resting right now, and he doesn't need any visitors."

Teasingly—I know he was teasing—he took his name tag and said, "This says I can go anywhere I want to."

So I took my name tag and said, "This says registered nurse, and you're not going in my patient's room."

Well, he went back and told the board and others that I refused to allow him to go see the patient. He was so proud of the fact that we were protecting the patient and it didn't matter who wanted to visit. They were not going in.

When this executive and his wife were told that he had cancer of the spine, they were holding each other and crying and trying to work through that process. A physician who was a personal friend came to visit. I was standing outside the door; I had closed the curtain and the door. He came to the door and said I need to go see them.

I said, "Not right now."

He said, "I happen to be a good friend of theirs."

I said, "I happen to be the nurse, and you're not passing through this door." He got mad and left. When he came back later, he apologized when he went in. They told him, "We're so proud that he did that."

This is a first-class operation. The focus is on taking care of total joints. The nurses are wonderful; they are so conscientious, and because they don't float, we work with the same team every day, time after time. They have become the best surgery assistants I've worked with, and that's key. When nurses are not familiar with a procedure, it takes more time. These nurses are aware of what's going on. The Joint Replacement Center is really a smooth system, and it works well. This means less stress on all of us. This makes for happy people, happy patients. It's a real team atmosphere.

On this unit, I find recovery time for my patients is quicker; in fact, sometimes I have to slow them down. The Joint Replacement Center team is the best from a physician's point of view. We just have to mention, "It sure would be nice if . . ." and the next thing you know, the staff on the floor make it happen. All the red tape is gone. Everyone is empowered to make things happen.

New Employees

Our orientation program is outstanding; our training team put it together. It is experiential and designed so that people know we want to give patients the kind of care they'd like to give to their family. Everyone knows what that means for the hospital by the time orientation is over. Then we trust them to do what they came here to do.

I use a letter from a patient during new employee orientation. This patient talks about all aspects of patient-centered care, and I read it to let people know about it from the patient's point of view. I tell them that this is how we need to be. I go through several stories. I also have a video that I show of people here that have done things that have helped each other, helped patients, or helped their families.

When I go into an orientation session, I'm very hopeful when I give the introduction to standards. I am thinking 95% of what I'm going to say is so true, and 5% is what I want to be true. I think we have to paint a picture for the team members that we are a loving organization come what may. So every time I go in to talk to a new group, my thought is, "I've got to make sure I come across very sincere," and typically I do because I am. It needs to be personal to them. So as I am talking I try to gauge their receptivity. If I start to lose them, then I do things to draw them back into the conversations. I call on them and say, "What do you think about this?" or walk around the room and bring them back in.

When I draw my organizational chart for people in this organization, I say it's an upside-down triangle. I'm at the bottom, with patients and front-line caregivers at the top. My role is to be a supportive, resource-gathering leader. We also talk about how important I believe it is that we are clear in articulating our intentions. You know your intentions, and I know mine; however, people can only judge you by your actions. So, for me, one of the challenges in leadership is to make your intentions and your actions come ever closer and closer together.

We are quality from the ground up, and you can't argue with success. We have the highest marks around the hospital. We recruit people interested in succeeding. We are involved from the start with sharing our needs. Doctors wanted something more efficient. We got a lot of principles from other hospitals by going out and getting a program and then looking at it carefully. We selected one that had been successful, and we made a real commitment to making it a success here. Interviews for the jobs were held. No one just got put on the unit; you had to be selected to work there. Everybody here is on board and committed to the concept. I tip my hat to the hospital.

You had to apply to be on the Joint Replacement Center. To work there you had to be enthusiastic, share the same vision, and have the same goals as the team. You had to want the whole team to be successful. We did sort of a pattern interview, and we let the applicants share their stories. The unit was and still is a very successful unit. It is different than the rest of the units. It was the only unit for an entire year that had zero turnover in nursing, which is unheard of.

Doing It Better

The difference is that the hospital has empowered people to make decisions, and the people want to make it right. It took commitment and letting go from the top to let this work. It is complimentary, and it has improved outcomes. The length of stay has shortened because patients do take ownership of their own care and the staff partners *with* them. The patients do a heck of a lot better before and after surgery. Speed of recovery is better.

They also measure our successes and they let us know about them. We have team goals and expectations that are a part of the overall goals for the hospital. They turn over how we achieve those goals, and let us decide. We get measurements sent to us monthly so that we know whether what we are doing is working. The poster on our wall says, "90% customer satisfaction," and we haven't had any staff turnover now in 2 years.

We were missing the mark meeting an indicator of the criteria. I recognized that we had a deficiency. So, what we did was we got together, the manager and I. We would come in and redo the order sets for the physicians. We involved the staff, and every day, every shift we had to check the time, the surgery in-time. It was a huge undertaking. It's a continuous all-day thing.

The expectation is that we will be 100%, and we've been 100% for four months in a row now; however, that's just a known thing you have to do, and you constantly have to be aware of it.

Sometimes we feel like if we get something wrong we are going to be in trouble. There is not punishment, but we strive to be a service unit of excellence;

we do stand out in the hospital. The community comes to our units. We are featured on the website. We won the President's Award for quality, and we were recognized again this year for holding the gains. So, we just know that we have to be a little better. It puts a lot of stress on us because we are not the best; however, we are pretty darn good, and we know that. It makes us want to do better, constantly just doing a little better at all times. So, we just have to stay heightened, and our awareness has to be heightened.

Soul Stories

I have a little lady I want to tell about—my lady is 8. She was in an auto accident and had a small bleed in her head. She came in on nights, and I took care of her the next day and subsequent days. She was such a character. With her head injury, she was not on a ventilator; it wasn't significant enough for that. She was dazed and confused and had several lucid moments and some not so lucid.

One of the things I remembered was that she had the most beautiful blue eyes. One of the first times she was getting out of bed, I told her, "Don't look at the ground. It makes you dizzy; pick a point to look at." She would look right at me, right at my eyes, and we would move her to do the things she needed to do. She became very dependent and close to us as a result.

She had a very close-knit family. She did very well and was discharged home. I gave the family one of my cards and told them to let me know how she's doing. I wanted to hear.

A week after she was discharged I got a call at home about 9:30. She had been home and had gone to the bathroom and tried to get up. She fell and hit her head on the washing machine, and they were bringing her to the hospital. They had called to ask me if there was anything they could do. I told them, "Let me just come and see her." So I came and saw her in the ER that night, and she had a second bleed, a major bleed. It was unsurvivable. We took care of her and were able to get her into hospice. She lived for two weeks in hospice.

They took her home, and I went to visit several times. She had a bed set up in the living room. The family was surrounding her bed, and they laughed. They joked. They played. That was the thing about this family that impressed me. It wasn't all just sorrow and grief; it was joy. This family was extraordinary. They were so supportive of each other. I looked at this lady lying in the bed totally comatose and felt somewhat jealous—she was surrounded. What better can you have? When she died, her family was surrounding her bed.

The lady had a daughter who made plaster casts of her hands before she passed. It was one of those things that could cause chills up your spine. She made one for her niece and each one of her children so that they could have their mother's hands.

Early one Sunday morning, we were told we were getting a trauma patient coming in from North Carolina. It was a vehicle accident. The gentleman was killed, but they brought his fiancé up. She was on a ventilator, and we were getting the patient settled in and everything. The doctor came and talked to us, and he said, "Keep her alive until we can get her momma here."

We couldn't find her mother; we really didn't know who this little girl was, and it broke all of our hearts to see this beautiful girl lying here. We got her driver's license and started calling everybody. We called a friend that works for the police department and told them, "This girl is from North Carolina, and you need to find somebody. The doctor has told us she's not going to make it."

Someone found her parents, and when they got here, they were the most loving momma and daddy that ever were. Her momma and daddy fell in love with all of us. They were very dependent on us. The doctors came in and wanted to do something. The parents came to us and asked, "Is it okay?" They wouldn't accept what the doctors were telling them unless they were getting affirmation from us that they were doing the right thing.

From the beginning of her arrival, of course, I am talking to her. We talk to our patients like they are going to answer us back at anytime. I said, "Can you hold up two fingers for me?" All of sudden she held up two fingers. Well, we were on cloud nine! When she woke up she didn't know who I was, but she knew my voice. She told us that she could hear everything that was ever said to her. She was our Christmas gift. We got her little gifts and a stocking and put a little Christmas tree in her room. She eventually went home.

We have a harpist who is a medical intern at East Tennessee State University. She comes routinely and plays for patients. One day she stopped into a room where an older woman was dying. The patient hadn't responded to anyone in several days. The old woman's daughter was with her when the harpist came in and offered to play for them. As the harpist played, the comatose woman raised her arm, although she did not open her eyes or engage in any other way. The daughter took her mother's hand and held it while the harpist played. When the music stopped, the old woman's arm went down. Her daughter turned to the harpist and said, "Now I can let go."

We had an older man on the intensive care unit floor, and his cardiovascular system was shutting down; we knew it was just a matter of time. He loved basketball, and his team, Illinois, was playing in March Madness. His son asked to stay with him so that they could watch March Madness together. The nurse was adamantly opposed; she felt it would be too stressful on his heart. The rest of the intensive care unit team and the patient advocate, however, met with her and shared their conviction that loving care for a patient in his condition was to allow it. She reluctantly agreed to let the son stay.

The patient and son watched the game, and Illinois won that year; it was such an important moment for them. Several weeks later the man died, and the son expressed his deepest gratitude for the staff's willingness to bend the rules. This year when March Madness rolled around that nurse told all of us, "I'm so glad we let them have that time together; his son will have a wonderful last memory with his dad."

It took awhile for all the nurses to come around to seeing why it was important to do that, especially in ICU, but with teamwork and our commitment to the patient first, we have 100% on board. Visitation for patients needs to be flexible.

I've learned to always look with my heart and be understanding with my patients. There was this little old man with a broken hip on my floor. Medically he was given only partial clearance for surgery, but he chose to have the operation anyway since he probably would have died without the hip replacement. He was appreciative of our care, but just a grumpy, unpleasant person to be around. I could have reacted to his irritability, but instead, I thought, "He could be my grandfather and he's hurting," and that allowed me to give him loving care. I had spent time with him, came immediately when he called, took care of his needs, and responded to his emotional needs. He never changed. He was grumpy until the day he left. When he was ready to go, he grabbed my arms and with determination brought me close enough so that he could kiss me on the check, and he whispered, "Thank you." I could tell he really cared, and it brought tears to my eyes. His daughter gave me a hug; it just felt like taking care of family. I make a difference here!

The Unexpected

Members of the Johnson County community are our volunteer musicians. We have a grand piano in the entry lobby, and occasionally, I will take a break and play or we have professional performances. A harmonica player comes weekly and tours the hallways, asking patients who are alone if they'd like a song. A maintenance man from a local church travels the corridors and plays guitar for patients. A vocalist comes weekly and does the same thing. She has a beautiful voice. One day I walked by, and she and a patient were singing a hymn together. I just had to stop and listen. It sounded beautiful.

The sweetest sound I have ever heard come out of this place was when I had a patient and he was going to die. He had a big bleed, and he was going to die. He sang with a choir in church, plus he was also in a quartet. He had been in this quartet for years. The family came to me and said, "There's some members of the choir out here, and they would love to sing with him one more time."

Of course, me, you know, I say, "Okay." I opened the doors of his room; I know there were 30 people. I didn't care. Anyway, they all went in, and I said, "I am going to shut the curtains and the door; you all go ahead and sing to him." The next thing you know it was like what you always think of when angels sing.

I wanted to get some true feedback from the physicians on what we can do to improve our facility. I wanted to get a feel for how they feel about leadership. I met with one doctor, and I asked, "How would you like me to communicate with you?" The doctor said, "I would like to have breakfast with you." So I had my secretary call him up, and we set up a time for breakfast and sat down and talked.

First of all, I wanted to get to know him, and I wanted him to get to know me. We needed to know each other better. I wanted him to tell me how we can do a better job. Was there anything I could do personally to make his job easier—anything we could do as a hospital that would make this an easier place for him to practice medicine? Were there any services or anything that he needed that we are missing out on? Were we helping him practice more efficiently, or were we being a hindrance in doing that? So I was trying to get him to talk to me and give me the information I needed so that I'd be able to give him a better place to practice. Hopefully he would get to know me better so that we would have a better working relationship.

At the same time, he had some things that he wanted to talk to me about. He wanted to start an infertility clinic, and he asked if I had enough time to talk about that. Since that time, over the past three or four months, we've been able to get what he wanted set up. So if I hadn't done this, I wouldn't have had that information.

Believing in People

I see my role as more of a shepherd of other folks. For example, let's say you asked a question and there are two of us in the room; I could answer you, but that other person in the room might be more perfect to answer because it's his area. He needs to shine in that area. Say you asked about physicians. I could say, "This is what we do for physicians and this is how we do it," and I certainly know all that; however, another person in the room would be the person who does that on a daily basis. So as a shepherd, I would prefer for them to be able to share their story. A good example is when we had our site visit for the Baldrige Award. When a question came for area X, if they looked to me first, I would say, "So and so would be the most appropriate person to answer, as his role in the organization is X." It tells the person asking the question that this is the person who is really responsible for this area. It also tells the person who is responsible that you have faith in them in what they do.

I'm the one who has to set the tone and set the expectations. We've had a couple of retreats, and at one retreat, we spent two days on how to say "thank you." That may seem a little odd, but there are lots of people that have never said thank you. They don't know how to write a thank you note. My expectations were that they would write thank you notes. At first I think some people thought it was corny, but now we see more notes around here, some even sent to me. When I see someone doing something positive, I jot down their name, and I look them up to find out where they work. I send a note that says something nice about them. I write several notes every day.

I try to send thank you notes either to work or home to thank people for very specific actions: thank you for doing X on this date. This is what it meant to us. If you send it to his or her home, then everyone at home gets to celebrate it. Also, most of us get mail, but it's just another bill. When you get letters at home, however, you say, "What's this?"

They are always handwritten. I keep note cards in my car and keep them at the desk. I try to every week send somebody a note so that we are continuing to validate employees and people. I keep them in the car and just write them at stoplights because oftentimes you mean to do this but you don't get them done. I find myself on the road in between places a lot, and you can write notes driving down the road. When I come back, I can ask to please mail these out. Our department did a wonderful job of developing a database for me where everybody in the organization can have their home addresses loaded into a database for thank you notes. On this database, I can also jot down why

I sent the note. So, if I sent you a note two months ago, I might put in there. The next time I'm thinking I need to write you a note, I can pull that up and say, "Well, gosh it's been four or five months since I've written him a note. That's not very good of me." So, it's a good tool for us just to keep us motivated in that direction.

The other thing is you have to have happy employees or team members if you want to have happy patients. So, one way that we build morale with our team members is by acknowledging them for good work, and hopefully, they will pass that good feeling on to the people they are caring for. We all write thank you notes. My wife showed me a note that she received when she was in the hospital with chest pains. She had to spend the night to have tests done. She got a note from the nurses on the floor afterward, and each nurse had written a personal note inside it.

They are good people. One of the people who reports to me was having a really, really bad day, but she had accomplished so much. I thought that she was being hard on herself. She wasn't recognizing how successful she had really been. I wanted her to know that she has such great potential in a leadership role and that even though during this particular episode she felt beaten up on, that when looking at everything about her, she is ragingly successful—what she does that makes my life easier and makes me look good. I just sent her some flowers and a little card that said, "Thank you so much for the difference you make. You are so helpful to me."

We have so many stories that tell people what we expect. For example, one of our patient care attendants was taking care of a man that was homeless. He didn't have any shoes when he came in, and he was getting ready to go home. She gave him her shoes: He went home with shoes, and she went home barefoot. We spotlight loving care no matter where it is given.

Another example happened during the wintertime. An employee came outside, and her car wouldn't start. Another employee came out, and even though he lived here, he took her all of the way to Kentucky, where she lives. That's an employee helping another employee. That's how I try to build a culture within the organization of caring and love.

We sent out a survey, and I responded to every one of them. First of all, I hand wrote a note. I think it's very important that people know that you take the time to read their feedback. I think that a lot of physicians probably felt like this was going into a big hole somewhere and that they would never hear anything back from it. So I wrote a note and thanked them for returning their questionnaire and for the positive things that they had to say about the hospital. I told them about those people whose lives were made better while they are at the hospital. I also mentioned that I had also written that person a note to let them know how much they thought of them. I know that they'll appreciate knowing that because a lot of times people don't get that pat on the back.

For example, I sent one person a note and let her know that a physician had commented that she was a person who had been very special to him. I just wanted to pass on that positive feedback and to let her know that I'm proud to have somebody like her on our team. Then I sent a note to the doctor telling him what I did and my appreciation of his sharing the feedback about a staff member. If there are any comments about things we need to improve, I'll address that in the note, too. I let them know I'm going to look into their concerns and will follow-up with them. Everybody needs a pat on the back. That's the kind of culture I've been trying to develop here, a positive culture where we tell people that we care about them and show people that we care about them.

People have to believe in you and that you do what you say you are going to do. If I make a mistake, I don't mind letting people know; I will always tell people. I had one boss who always told us, "If you don't make any mistakes, you're not doing anything."

One day I showed up for surgery, and someone outside of the unit had scheduled surgeries without consulting the floor. It just should not have happened. The next morning when I walked into the hospital I was met by the hospital administrator who apologized for what had happened the day before. He assured me that the staff on the floor had not known either and that the communication mix up had been cleared up and that it would never happen again, and it hasn't. Can you imagine an administrator meeting me like that? It is unheard of for an administrator to apologize for something like that, much less meet you at the front door as you walk in. I am just so impressed with their commitment here.

On one night shift I had 6 or maybe 10 people in a meeting, and we were going through a rough time. Morale was low, and we were going through just a bumpy time. Two of the nurses mentioned that they were unhappy and potentially going to leave. I thought I'd better do something. I said, "Let's talk about this." They were both from out of town, and I said, "You've come here. You've worked here a year. Let's talk a little bit more about why you're here.

What keeps you here? What's going to keep you here? Is it the money? Is it the hospital? What is it?" One of the nurses said, "I really like this facility. I like the people that I work with. I like the doctors. Even though it's a level 1 trauma center, it doesn't feel like it. I don't know how long I will be able to stay here, but I would like to stay here because of what you all stand for." She did like our vision of constantly seeking out and doing innovative things, going that extra mile, and our patient-centered care philosophy. That's our main focus here in Mountain States—just patient-centered care. I knew that by keeping that in their mind and at the forefront and keeping them focused on why they stay, why they're here, and why they chose nursing, was important.

After I heard their story, you know I listened to them, and I told them my story. So we sort of shared the commonalities between ourselves, and I sort of gave them a pep talk. I said, "It's not always great. I don't always love my job. Nobody always loves his or her job. If they say they do they are probably lying because everybody has bad days. Some people throw the towel in quicker than others, but everybody thinks about it some time. Is it really worth it?" Those nurses are still here by the way, still very happy, and I could have lost them two times since then, but they still share that same vision. One has come over to the other one's way of thinking; they have become really good friends. I think just sharing what is important to us and what we want to do for our patients is really what's kept them here. It's not the money. It's just the camaraderie.

Work Family

I enjoy people, and I do so I enjoy coming to work. It helps when you like the people you work with. I am appreciated, and they tell me that. Everyone is helpful, and nobody talks bad about you.

Her son has been hospitalized in a mental facility for various things, and this has really been a stressor for her family. Having been a parent for a long time you can really relate to some of the things that are going on in her world. I think we all have internal things that have happened to us that are distressful and you are trying to outwardly balance everything. I mean I could feel her pain. I know the distress of being a parent, trying to do the best you can, and sometimes it takes different detours. So just an empathetic listening ear, support for what she was going through, and then also just helping her to know that we recognize it and know that it's impacting her right now are important.

We've adjusted some of her hours, the times that she actually comes in. She's an early-bird kind of person. Right now we are doing a lot of program development, protocols, and orders and order sets and all of those kinds of things. So a lot of what she's doing right now just requires work and tasks, but it doesn't have to be done from 9 to 5 or 8 to 4 or whatever. So she's coming in like at 5:00 a.m., which is by her choice. It works with her schedule because they are going to counseling sessions. She knows that she can come in and get her work done. We report off on that. We look to see what are the targets, what's going on, and then she can still get to her counseling sessions, do what she needs to do with that. Right now I think we are balancing that pretty well because we are still getting things accomplished and we are staying on course while still providing a listening ear. So it's a balance between the two.

She just came in to my office as I was leaving one day and said, "Have I told you today that I love my job?"

I said, "That's good to hear." She is being encouraged on the professional side, which she sees as a reward, which I think right now is also balancing out some of the distress she is feeling on the personal side. So, as a parent, she is feeling like there are less than successful stories happening right now, but she is seeing that we are making the steady improvement and accomplishments through the stroke department and that's been a positive for her.

I'm just a little different in my approach to my staff. We don't shy away from not getting involved in our employees' personal lives. Some are better than others. I'm probably more assertive than others in the way that I'll stop and ask, "How are you feeling? How's your mom?" I know all of my employees' children's names. I know what they're doing, what sport they play. It's really important to know that. It was important to me when I was on the floor working—for my manager to know about me. I try to stay involved with my employees' personal lives outside because it's reality. You spend a lot of time here with each other, and this is an extended family. So I try to recognize that.

We have seen this unit grow from a small unit to a state-of-the-art facility. The facilities are the top of the line, and administration is supporting this. There is a sense of community that we have as nurses. We are a tight-knit group, and we are brothers and sisters. We love one another. We laugh together. We work hard together. We cry together. We pray together. We share our experiences. We share our patients, and we support and love one another. This allows us to provide an environment where the family knows that any need can be asked of any one of us. They know that need will be met and provided for until their nurse becomes available. The community supports the nurses; this provides us the opportunity to customize the care that a patient demands. It's about personal relationships. We adopt them and they adopt us.

Before we moved into the intensive care unit, we were stocking it. One of the night shift nurses said, "We need to do something as a group before we move into this unit. We need to have a blessing for the unit." We met in the waiting room; it was quiet before the hustle and bustle, and one of the staff led that blessing. We had prayer, blessed us and blessed the unit before it opened. It created the space.

It will never, ever be a quiet space again. It was so awesome; you could hear a pin drop. We knew we were embarking on a new journey so special, and you had all of these feelings from folks that you knew you would be and want to spend time with. It bonded us even more. We took ownership of one another, through love and support and holding each other accountable. It went beyond just co-worker connection. It went to heart connection.

Have you ever worked with anybody where you knew there was something you needed to go take a look at? You have a feeling you need to go into a room, but it is not your patient. It's like you know you needed to be there— your co-worker needed you. It's like when women know their child is in trouble. When we work together so long, we know when the other is in trouble. I have been standing by many a time when I was getting ready to yell and someone walks into the room saying, "I was just checking to see what was going on in here." We have that electricity that pulls you to them.

Seizing the Moment

We're not just good to our patients; we treat one another with loving care also. We nicknamed one of our nurse directors the *Queen of Notes*. She sends notes of recognition, thanks, encouragement, praise, and congratulations. You name it, and she sends it—to everyone, not just employees.

I noticed an announcement in the newspaper regarding this nurse who had recently passed a special certification, and I sent her a congratulations note for her achievement. I didn't think much more about it. Much later I was interviewing a nurse for a position on a unit here at the hospital. During the interview the nurse said, "You don't remember me do you? You were the only person who sent me a note after my certification, and that really made an impression on me. When I saw this opening and saw that you were a part of the program, I knew I wanted to be a part of it too."

We do a great job trying to assist our families with what they need, especially at the time when someone is going to die. I don't know why, but one night, I got called in to work on the night shift. I found out later why it was. A friend of ours that we worked with, his sister was brought in here with a drug overdose. She had years and years of problems, and just so happened she was assigned to me. She had a daughter who was 14 years old. Because her mother had a long hard time with drugs, this girl pretty much raised her mother. There was a younger brother, and she had also taken care of him. The mother was pretty much gone, and the girl came to me and said, "There is one thing I'd like to do. Before my mother leaves me, I'd like to just lay down with her one more time."

I said, "Everybody out of the room. I'll call you back in just a little while." I moved her mother over and got her a pillow. I patted the bed and said, "Come on over here." She climbed in that bed with her momma, and I went out. I dared anyone to go in that room until the girl called.

After about an hour of being with her mom, she came out and said, "I can do it now." I got a card from her later telling me what that hour meant to her. So it's things like that we do on a daily basis to try to help with not only the needs of the patient but the needs of the family, too. That is something that girl will always remember, something that will never go away. It was something special that she needed, just her and her mother. I think we do this daily.

I make rounds periodically in the hospital, and I don't make them every day because some days I am in meetings all day. While I was making rounds, I stopped at the nursing station to see how everything was going, if they had all the equipment and things they needed. This was the nursing station that we just reopened. While I was up there, I found out that there were a couple of things that were left out, like a lamp tray. So I called our guy who is head of materials management, and I told him. He went down to the store about 9:00 o'clock that night and came back and brought a tray that would work because we didn't have any in the hospital. So he took the initiative after I talked to him to get those people what they needed.

Coaching and Being Coached

My intentions are to never come off as being a boss. So that's one of the things that I ask her. When you see me doing things that you say, "Wait a minute. I think there's a gap here between intentions and actions." I need you to tell me that. So I can say, "You know, you're right. What I intended was not this action. There was a gap there." So anytime we're in a meeting together either at our regular mentoring sessions or some other time just on the fly, we will do a debriefing, and I will tell her how I thought she did. She will tell me how she thought I did. I'll say frequently, "We've got one business folks—it's the patient in the bed. How will the decision we are about to make affect the patient in the bed?"

The nurse was an intern at the time. She was a nursing student and in her senior practicum. I could see so much potential in her, but she was very withdrawn. I guess she was not a people person. She has evolved since into that. I had her for two semesters, and then she became a management student of mine. She just did not have any self-esteem, but I saw a great potential in her. She had thought about just getting her two-year degree, and I said, "No, you need to go. You're in it. You need to keep going."

She was like, "No, no."

I said, "Yes, yes, you are going. We will get you tuition reimbursement here. We will make sure that we work with your schedule. We will get the time off that you need. We will get you a preceptor. We will do the whole thing." So I convinced her to do so.

After a couple of years, she finished her school. She is now in her fourth year here as a senior primary nurse. She is my head nurse on my unit. Still, at times, she second guesses herself. I have to remind her of where she was, where she came from, and what all she's accomplished. I remind her to stop and celebrate moments that have happened to her and to reflect back on and remind her of where she's at in life. She's very successful. Her peers very much respect her. She is becoming a wonderful leader, and probably in a few more years, she'll be at the point to where she could really go into management. She is going in the right direction. She's involved in a lot of our councils here at the hospital. In fact, she was just the only nurse that was selected to go to a particular conference. She got a very prestigious award last year.

I saw her potential just by the way that she interacted with her patients. I would go in oftentimes, and she would be sitting on the end of the bed. That's a lost thing nowadays because we are short staffed and very busy. Patients are sicker. There are constraints on how long you can stay here. So you just get caught up in the busyness and sometimes, somehow, we leave that human touch part out. So I would find her sitting on the bed or sitting there holding a patient's hand while they were talking. She was doing more than she really needed to be doing at the level she was in her career and in school, but she always had the initiative to do things. She always had good ideas, but I sort of had to pull it out of her. Over the past few years, she has just really come out of her shell. She's gotten married, something that she said she'd never do. She's coming around. She's really blossomed into a nice, young lady. I'm very proud of her.

We give people constant positive feedback. We acknowledge their work when they are achieving success. In fact, we discovered that people don't really know how to say thank you in very many ways, so we addressed that; education is very important for us. We responded by creating a seminar on how to say thank you. We put together a *tool box* for leaders that included star cards, thank you notes that had the words "Nothing Other than Excellent Service" on the front, movie passes, small gift items, and a book we'd composed with 365 ways to give feedback for excellence. We even included sprigs of rosemary that they could enclose in their notes. Rosemary is associated with remembrance. Adding a touch of something fragrant was an added touch that really said "thank you" with more meaning.

I am a Baldrige examiner. So, I know what criteria they are looking for. I am able to listen to what others say and how they answer the question and make suggestions. I am more like a safety net listening for what answers are coming out and making sure we share out entire story.

We met with a Baldrige consultant in the boardroom. There were five or six folks there. Three people were really on target; one person was really not on target at all. The challenge was to take the person who wasn't on target and allow that person to be successful and feel validated.

On the one side you are thinking, "Oh, hush. We've got to move on." On the other side you are thinking, "How can we get from there to here?" From my perspective, I don't care what the issue is. You never want to publicly take someone and say they are wrong. You want to take what they're doing and channel them to the right direction. So I spent a portion of my time listening for what they were saying, what were the nuggets in there that they are saying, and how can we move those nuggets into what we are really looking for. At the conclusion of the meeting, after everybody had gone home, one of the positive comments was, "You did a good job today. I watched you, and I noticed that you were trying to bring so and so back on task." That told me that we were probably getting the right thing accomplished.

One mentoring meeting stands out for me was when I said to her, "You know, I need us to be able to talk about your goals and objectives, what you hope to get out of our mentoring relationship."

She said to me, "I constantly hear throughout the hospital what a wonderful leader you are, and I want to learn what you do that makes that so." So we had a great time sitting down at Panera Bread talking about her goals and objectives and how she believed I could help her. I talked about how I was certain she could help me.

I know where my shortcomings are, and I've worked on them. I know where some of my blind spots are about how good I am, but don't really even think about it. The only way I'm going to get better in my leadership style is for you to tell me what you see. Tell me how I can become a better leader for you. When we do our performance reviews I say, "When you schedule with me, I want you to bring two measurable ways in which I can become a better leader for you." I get some great ideas.

It's very easy to surround oneself with people like oneself, but I believe that diversity in a leadership team is extremely critical. So I hired a different personality type for a director position. It was really a struggle. The first time we did a review she said, "It absolutely drives me crazy when you come late to a meeting."

I said, "Thank you for telling me that because I can control that." I will consciously make a decision. Do I stay in the meeting I'm in and finish it up and then be late for the next one, or do I excuse myself and come meet with you? That's the choice I will make. It's because you have told me what your needs are in me as a leader. That's great. I love to learn about me, and I love to make changes. My intention is to become the best leader I can possibly be, and I know I've got a lot to learn.

I set the tone and the expectations. If I tell people I want them to go out and make rounds and they don't see me out making rounds, then they know I'm not living up to what I want them to do, and my personal philosophy is I work for everybody here. If I were putting people on the organizational chart, I would be at the bottom holding everybody up. My goal is to help provide them support, provide them the tools to work with, other people to work with; I'm the lowest man on the totem pole.

Going Out of the Way

I remember one night I had already gone home after work. I heard the helicopters overhead, and I knew they were headed to the ER. So I got in my car and drove over there to see if they needed anything. There had been a terrible, multicar accident, and I knew the staff was going to be there all night. I checked in with the doctors and nurses to see what they might need. I stopped and talked with folks in the waiting area to let them know what was happening and that there were so many emergencies that they were going to have to be patient. It may not have been the right thing to do for our census, but I even told one person that there was a much shorter wait time at one of the other hospitals. On the way back home, I was about to pass a Krystal's restaurant. I thought about my crew, and instead of driving home, I turned in and ordered 60 Krystals to go. I drove them back to the hospital for the nurses and doctors that were working behind the scene.

There's one slide that shows an older lady who was dying and had no family. The nurses had turned the bed in ICU to face the mountains, and they were rubbing her head, holding her hand, letting her know that she wasn't alone. We had our harpist, who is the wife of one of our doctors, that was up there playing music. That's how we encourage our folks to go out of the way.

I am the CEO, but I like to buy bears for a lot of older people. It's something I just think about. The little man I was telling you about that was dying the same time my father was. He was another older man, about 90 years old. I went up to see him, and he had a little bibbed overalls lying in the bed. He was so happy about dying because he felt like he was going to another place where he wouldn't be suffering. He was really happy, so I went and got him a bear.

I might stop in and ask patients how they're doing. Has your service been good? Is there anything I can do personally to help you? I would be happy to do whatever you need. I bought a teddy bear for one little lady who was just a sweet, kind little lady. She still could smile a little bit. I went back up to see her the next day, and her bear was over by the window. Somebody had taken it and moved it. I went and got her bear and put it back over by her, and she just hugged it. Little things like that mean a lot to people.

Editor Commentary

This is an inspirational story about telling and retelling inspirational stories! Mountain States Health Alliance has tapped into a most powerful way to unite their staff and help them to understand how they can (and do) make an incredible difference to their patients, families, visitors, and the community. The concept of "loving care" could potentially appear "hokey," but staff members at all levels embrace it as more than a slogan, but as an aspiration.

This simple statement "loving care" and the stories that are told as a result serve to teach and remind the staff of their ability to make a difference to each individual patient and family member. There were dozens of stories of how employees translated this into making a decision to do something unique for a patient—whether watching the Illinois basketball game or having the church choir sing for a patient. Staff members can clearly articulate how this power to make a difference translates into a higher level of engagement, teamwork, pride, and satisfaction for them.

The leadership at Mountain States has taken an unyielding approach to excellence in all facets of their organization. There is no complacency. They are constantly challenging their employees and physicians to "push the envelope" in all aspects of their operations. They ask constantly, "What are the metrics? How can we do better?" It's an approach based on recognizing that there is a lot of good already being done and that the employees can build on what is already going well to do even better.

The means by which they accomplish this is to bring out the best in the employees by engaging both their hearts and minds. Leaders ensure that the stories are captured and communicated—told and retold—and used as examples for recognition and for learning. In turn, this leads to the creation of even more extraordinary moments—a positive, upward spiral.

The leaders appear extraordinarily self-aware that what they do is as important as what they say. They set the example of the vision of the organization and role model the expected behaviors. They practice what they preach. Their self-criticism (I am getting better at this) gives permission for employees to have the courage to ask this question of themselves. Getting better is not to be feared, but rather embraced.

Reward and recognition are used in abundance, and thank you notes are used liberally. The managers have the tools to create a variety of types of recognition and are expected to use them. The leaders take the time to show their appreciation for the employees and their special efforts to make a difference. The employees feel appreciated (and noticed) for their efforts, and their hearts are encouraged to continue to perform at this level.

Stories are powerful tools—as inspiration, aspiration, and affirmation. Mountain States has taken story telling to a high level. The leaders have honed their skills of encouraging the hearts and minds of their employees by living the values, teaching the values, developing expectations around the values, and celebrating (with enthusiasm and often) when others are living them as well.

Table 9-1   Organizational Demographics

Organization	The Cathedral Foundation of Jacksonville, Inc.
Location	Jacksonville, FL
Setting	Urban
Communities served	Urban
Type of organization	Organization serving older persons through housing and community services
Number of FTEs	280
Focus area	Cathedral Gerontology Center, Inc.
Focus area served	Affordable senior housing, Meals on Wheels, Community Care for the Elderly, Protective Counseling Services, Guardianship Education, Nursing Home Diversion
Focus area	Center for Medicare and Medicaid Services (CMS)
Best practices and awards	2004 Champion Award presented by FMQAI in recognition of NHAQI Remarkable Achievement
	No agency use in 7 years
	Host facility for community colleges for nursing students, pharmacy students, and administrator-in-training programs

CHAPTER 9

Lead or Get Out
of the Way

The stories in this chapter are the voices of the corporate CEO with the Cathedral Foundation, the administrator, the vice-president of nursing, and the medical director of the gerontology center, the staff of the gerontology center, the residents and their family members, and members of the Jacksonville, Florida community. Here are their stories.

THE CATHEDRAL FOUNDATION

The Future of Aging

"There was a big shift in the mid 1980s to focusing on seniors," the CEO states. We were good at taking care of elders. Then, in the late 1990s we came to recognize that the very thing we did in serving seniors was not something we wanted to age into. While we were really good at what we were doing, we realized, "If we were 72 and needed our services, this isn't what we would want."

That was a 6-month kind of heavy period for the foundation and for me personally. So the conversations we had shifted to, "What does it mean to grow older? What is it that we expect as we grow older? How does that inform the work that we do?"

We did an appreciative inquiry, and we explored the strengths and the future of aging. It was sort of like your own truth about aging. We did a couple hundred interviews. We looked at aging at its best, and we looked at our highest banners for service delivery. There was zero correlation. We realized that we were really good at the wrong job. This was another dark moment.

So then we began to explore, "How do we deliver on this." We began to look at aging from a position of strength. We recognized that even the global dialogue had demographic imperative. All aspects of aging had a marginalization to it, or even a fear. It wasn't simply the United States' marketing and ideas about aging. It was a global thing.

We then began to influence the global dialogue. We are preparing to launch the Center for Advanced Living, which will include global stories on the Internet that reinforces best practices in aging and informs responses to aging. We have explored "For the Love of Your Life" programs, and we've done some curriculum development.

The Cathedral Foundation itself is slated to be a research center. It has taken some awareness on the part of the board to shift from "doing for others" to "addressing the environment we age in." This doesn't mean abandoning our elders; it means adopting a completely different way of looking at who they are. This has become part of our conversations and our vocabulary at Cathedral. Our board travels to international conferences to gain insight in this area. We have an expectation of excellence and innovation. It is very challenging and very exciting.

The Nonmission

"Actually, I don't talk about mission, and this is a pretty big conflict with some of our board." When you state your mission in three cool words or five or ten words, you limit the possibilities. The mission statement in and of itself is a limiting belief. What I know is that if the staff connects to their purpose in life and they happen to do it here, why define that in terms of mission? Just celebrate their contribution.

I've never had a staff person say, "If you would just give me a mission statement, I could just change the world." If you are connected to your core purpose and you are in a setting where you can contribute your best effort, why we would frame that in any way but the gift that it is? It is richer on their terms than anything we can put on the back of a little card that they put in their wallet. Why would they use our words? It's the gift of their words. This is the hardest sell with my board.

We came to know our values and articulate them. They operate as reflections of the people in the organization. Prior to the process of discovering and excavating them, our values weren't brought up to the level of importance that they actually are.

So we do storytelling. In the storytelling, I ask people about their best moment with an elder or a family member or one another in the last year. As we move forward in the stories, we tease out what is at play. Then we honor that. It is like a confirmation that the DNA is the right DNA and it sort of strengthens the DNA for the time ahead. So it's interesting to me that although we don't have a values statement, when you are consistent with the stories and you pull the themes out, we have a generosity of spirit. We are resourceful and resilient. We have a kind of environment that extends not only to our residents but also to the community. In fact, you can actually see when we do things that are outside of our value core. Everybody knows when it's not right.

The Cathedral foundation is in line with who I am in terms of positive image, positive action. The Cathedral Foundation had hit the brick wall of efficiency: being routine, the excellence being routine. I said, "You know— almost anyone could run the Cathedral Foundation right now at this time." It is financially sound. Well, that doesn't hold anything. What I thought that conversation was preparing me for was to leave. This was maybe 10 to 12 years ago. Then we moved through the process of engaging the energy and momentum of the organization in a new way.

I read David Cooperrider's thesis (Positive Image, Positive Action) one night. A consultant had given it to me. It articulated what I was fuzzy about but knew to be true. I realized that our systems, whether it's our testing, our education, or our healthcare system, are all framed on the feedback of what's not working, but Cooperrider's idea of positive image and positive action was so wonderful. It was an affirmation that we really do gravitate toward the positive.

Partnerships

As the CEO of the Cathedral Foundation, I see unlimited potential for influencing the global society and the possibilities of aging. Then I see delivering it on a one-by-one basis whether it's with the elders or my employees. My personal belief is that "relationships" are all there is.

About five years ago I had a conversation with someone working at United Way about the fact that the way a community takes care of its elders is a reflection of the community health in its entirety. I thought United Way was not bringing leadership to that. So I thought, "Let's go to Vancouver for an international conference and begin to plug into the globalization of aging, its demographics and responses, and come up with some creative ideas."

As a result, The United Way made a 10-year commitment to explore aging at its best to create expectations for elders in volunteering. When they seized on it as the fundamental direction they would go, I'd have to say I was pretty surprised. I was amazed that I was actually influencing possibilities at United Way. On one side of the coin you can say they took many of the things the foundation is talking about and did something with them.

It all needs to be done, and there's lots of room to get it done. I currently serve on the Bridging Elder Care Network Task Force, and it has been rewarding for me. My involvement has advanced and focused United Way's direction.

A senior physician leader states, "My son and I developed a company, not-for-profit, that basically would encourage students to participate in the lives of elder patients." So we set up this not-for-profit corporation with the idea that a lot of patients, specifically those that are in this building, don't have any money, and many don't have any family. Their resident rooms looked institutional. The idea was that these students would go out to different businesses and get some contributions from the corporate world. They would use the money on resources to change the resident rooms to make them look more homelike.

They bought quilts or chairs to put in the rooms to make it look like a home environment. They bought frames for pictures they have of family members and placed them in their rooms. So now the rooms are more home-like rather than institutional. The same students come in and read to the residents. They bought radios so that residents could hear some of their favorite songs. That generated a lot of joy for us. That probably was the biggest joy that I've had.

Seizing the Defining Moment

There is a seminal defining event for the Cathedral Foundation. It was in response to Hurricane Andrew in the early 90s. We live in Florida, so we anticipate hurricanes and storms, but because we live in Jacksonville, we rarely have a storm experience. When we learned of the devastation of Hurricane Andrew, everybody was sort of, "Whew, not us," and then, "Oh, my gosh, all of those elders in South Florida, what will we do?"

There was what I called a "hand wringing to action step." We weren't going to send bottled water or do a clothing drive. We were going to do something about the elders down there. Colleagues were calling to say, "These elders are going to die in these shelters if you don't come get them." There was a tremendous amount of fear and heartache from others, and all of those emotions were immediately transferable to me, the Cathedral leader, in conversations. It was like an absolute call to bring the best of who we are to that situation right away.

Whatever had rallied in me was contagious. I knew the conviction would move through. It wasn't so much that I would pull people to a vision. It would be that people would come to a place where their contribution created the vision.

So everyone in the organization—and I mean *everyone*—did something about Hurricane Andrew. We agreed to come together at 7:00 a.m. at the church, and we put all of these easel papers all of the way around the room. We talked about what we could do. Then we decided that what we could do would not be limited by the assumption of no resources or access to resources. We rallied, "This is what we can do, and we're going to be successful." It was the shared conviction, and the shared responsibility that was so powerful.

I needed transportation. So I called the Congressman's office, and I talked to his staff. I said, "I need a jet to go down and pick these seniors up and bring them up to Jacksonville." Speed was of the essence.

They replied, "Well, I'll have to move heaven and earth to do that."

I said, "Well, that's good enough. Let's get it done."

Ultimately, they never sent a plane. The Homestead runway was so damaged that they couldn't use it. We couldn't get the elders from where they were to any airplane more efficiently than actually picking them up with a bus. So we sent buses down and relocated 60 elders from South Florida. We sent a chaplain with the bus driver so that they could begin working through the emotional traumas.

They came with nothing. They had no clothes, and many had no IDs. We moved them into apartments that had been renovated and furnished and included all of the things that we could think of: stamps, envelopes, rubber bands, linens, and televisions. We did a city-wide and county-wide appeal on the television, and we got volunteers from Navy bases. They came in with trucks, and they loaded furniture. Our residents who lived at Cathedral Residences sorted the furniture. We had a resident buddy for each senior who was moved here. We got Spanish sponsors, and we got community buddies to help reestablish their banking and their doctors.

We wanted to have phone books here that so people could settle in. I wanted them to have long-distance cards so that they could call their families. I wanted phones installed for them so that their people would know where they were and so that they could get comfort however they could get it. Well, of course, all phone people were busy in South Florida restoring service. Still I told them, "I want it done by tomorrow. I am bringing in a busload of seniors tomorrow." They need to have telephones installed. So they did. I called the phone company and said, "I would like for you to give me cards for these 60 seniors." They told me that they have to get approval somewhere. I said, "If you have to do that, then I have to call someone else." So I called someone else.

We took up office at the church. We had it like an operation center. Whatever people had a talent for doing, they did. Even if it was rounding up hangers from the dry cleaners so that people could have places to hang their clothes. The entire parish hall at the church was filled with clothing.

The woman that was in charge of the clothing was well into her 70s. She had heels on and had been on her feet the entire day. I said to her, "Please take a break or please wear more comfortable shoes." She told me that this was her business, her mission, and to please leave her alone to do it. It was an important lesson to me in trying to be helpful. When people are at their best, you need to just get out of the way.

Constancy of Purpose

One of the things I know is, the constancy of no matter what your contribution is, people believe you and support you. For many of our employees, this is the stability touchstone in their life. They may be single parents, or they may have transportation or financial issues. We are not the solution for all of those, but sometimes we are the respite from all of that. So I think constancy is a big part of it.

I believe people intend to do the right thing. When I interviewed a CNA, the woman told me her whole goal in life had been to become a CNA. She had arrived. I thought, "Gosh, we need to honor that." So it's sort of honoring the relationships and the constancy.

At Cathedral, there is a constancy. CNAs can pick up the phone and say, "We don't have enough staff to do what we are doing," or "this is not working." I don't know another nursing home where a CNA could call the CEO and know that she will listen to them and then do something about it.

We have great leaders at Cathedral. We are dealing with people who really understand. Here, character is a good thing. It's not about titles. It's not about who your husband is or how many diamonds you have. Character is important here and is not just built overnight.

When people say to me, "How is it that you have enough employees? We pay minimal tier wages in this community. So people ask, "How is it that you have enough staff?" I tell them that it is constancy; it is leadership.

When a new employee arrives, I will always tell them the ideal things we should do. We can give leeways if you make mistakes, but there are the things that we expect you to do. You will be accountable for that, but if at any time you are unable to fulfill this responsibility, you can always seek help from me. All that you have to do is ask. There are no stupid questions; there are just stupid actions.

I generally am in scrubs every day. I think the perception is that if you work, you understand my job, and you know what makes it work. So I don't mind getting out and working as a CNA, and you can't get out and work as a CNA in heels. So I'll wear scrubs and shoes that are comfortable every day. I'm there to help you turn a patient because I don't want you to come here complaining to me that it can't be done. It can be done.

A lot of times when you work for a company you never see the CEO—never. We see ours all of the time. She always has a hug. The administrator, she's the most caring person I know, and her caring is genuine. She listens. We call her Dr. Phil. This is my family. They make me feel like they care and love me, and that's great. I like working for Cathedral.

Engaging Staff

Our annual meetings for our board are simply story telling. What floats my boat is hearing the staff stories. I say, "Tell me your best moment about last year whether it was with a co-worker or with a patient." It takes a minute for anyone to speak publicly. I like the shyness before they get started. Then they leap into the story. The story connects with others, and you watch this contagious momentum. All of the stories are powerful. I've heard 300 stories in about six weeks. Afterward, there are board members that say, "I wanted to hear about your financial results."

I say, "Well, you can read."

I met with an all-hands meeting to announce that we don't have money for raises. Because of dramatically rising health insurance and electric bills and all of the other expenses, we are postponing a raise this year. The conversation opened up, and one woman said, "Just as you're feeling higher bills, I'm feeling higher bills too. What do you expect me to do?"

So I knew that in a healthy, family sort of way. People were going to grumble, but I also knew that we were going to be successful and that we would get to the place of trust. I was very aware of the energetics in the room. I wanted the steam or the pressure to happen there, rather than carried piece by piece into the work force and explode into little pieces. I acknowledged the person that had rising bills, just as the foundation has rising bills. I acknowledged that that was her reality. Rather than shutting that down, I was intentional about saying, "I understand that you are experiencing this."

Then one woman said, "You know. You're talking about health insurance, but the health insurance is not helping me and my four kids." This was a very unexpected development. We can do something about this. So I could feel myself thinking that this was going to come to a resolution.

The thing that stood out on that day was that as we began to trickle back to work or leave for the day, people began reassuring each other to trust the foundation. I overheard remarks like, "We can trust this. It's going to be fine."

At that meeting, we put together a coalition of people to look at different health care solutions. I asked them to do a survey of all the employees that worked here and asked them how their health insurance plan worked for them and if it could be different. We learned that some people had trouble with access to prescriptions. Some people had trouble with access to healthcare, and some people just want to be able to go to primary care. The coalition identified access to other community programs that would accomplish those employees' needs. Ultimately, we did give raises.

We celebrate with employees about their tenure or other specific accomplishments. We do that in small groups, and I do it all summer. When we come together as a group, another group is actually doing the breakfast or lunch for them. Some people are being celebrated, and other people are hosting. Throughout the organization, we do it that way.

Our CEO has a book club. It meets frequently because it is such a big project. There are 180 some-odd employees I think, and she has them all at her house in groups of six to nine. There is a common theme. Everyone is expected to go whether it's a housekeeper or a nurse. It is absolutely great. It makes everyone feel part of a whole.

With my boss there is always recognition. You might think she forgets, and at the end of the day, she will say, "Thanks you did a good job. I really appreciate it"—even if you are putting the trash out. She told me one time, "Why, you do the greatest job with the trash. I could never do it like you." So I had a big head all day.

I remember one day we had a real hectic day. I got a little gift card from my boss that said, "Thank you. I really appreciate you." She has this little thing that she always says that makes you feel special. She'll call you in your office. She has these little gift bags, and she will say, "Don't let anybody know I got it. It's just for you." Everybody has the same gift bag, but it's the way she presents it to you.

The Right Fit

I can take a tour with someone for five minutes, and I know if I want that person in this building. We may have worked together previously, and they were great. In this building, however, it may just not fit.

On the first interview, I walk with them around the building, and I go to all four floors. I purposely want to go where the residents are to see how the potential employee interacts with the other people that pass by. I want to see how they interplay with a family member, a volunteer, a resident, or whomever. I can tell by the way they speak to the residents, if they speak to the staff, if they touch them, or if they offer to help them. I can pretty much see if they are going to fit without them having to say a word. If they don't have the interaction and openness that I'm looking for well, there's no need to bring them back in for a second interview.

There was an unsuccessful administrator who hired an unsuccessful DON. Now both of those folks are probably successful where they are now, but they weren't successful here. They didn't come to lead. They came to work, be paid, and be boss.

Our new administrator was coming in to help get this place back on good footing. Her assumption was that everyone could be successful if they rose to the occasion, but her other assumption was that if they didn't rise to the occasion—in short order—they were out of here. I learned some things by witnessing this. The more accurately that she carved out the wrong people the more she actually upheld the right people.

When it was necessary to sort of re-establish discipline and to move people along who needed to go, it looked like too big a shift. I wanted to say, "Tone it down just a little bit. Take your time a little bit," but I knew the nursing home needed to be restored to excellence.

She came in when we needed to do carving out of the wrong influences and the wrong employees. We had to let nurses go that had been here a long time. We had to let CNAs go because their job contribution and their emotional energy were wrong for our organization.

There have been employees that I've let go. It's not a popularity contest. I may have liked them as an individual, but they did something that I was not willing to accept. I could see they were not part of the team that we wanted in the future. So you have to let them go, but I also always tell them that I don't fire anyone—they terminate themselves. I'm not saying that they were bad ones, but they weren't a good fit here with all of the changes that I knew would be taking place.

It is meaningful if it's six months later or eight months later for past employees to come back and say, "You were right. I have grown. I have strength. I have knowledge now, and I understand why you did what you did." It is meaningful that we are able to stay as friends and that they still respect me as a person and as a leader. I have two or three previous department heads that still do that.

We used agency staffing for about three months, and after that we eliminated it. Agency staff don't care about Cathedral the way our staff does. They say, "Hey, I'm getting a check. I'm out of here. I don't have to come back tomorrow and face these facts." So we decided agency staffing wasn't a good fit.

Some of our staff members have had to work a lot of overtime, but there was a lot of pride once we stopped using agency staff. We saw the nursing care turn around. We saw that our staff really loved the residents. They began to get them out of bed more often. They really began to nurture the residents, and things began to look better.

If I was leaving and I asked somebody to replace me, I would really want to see what that person was like because this is not just a job. This place is a very positive place. I wouldn't want somebody babysitting my kids unless I was comfortable with them. I would want to know who's coming into my home.

This job has been the perfect match for me. It's like I just stepped right into a place I've been all my life. Basically, it felt like everybody was very helpful and did whatever they could to help me to get acclimated to the organization. Everybody was right there for me.

I've been 27 years in various hospitals all over the country, and this was like a dream job for me—a dream place. The first thing the CEO does is "set you free." She says, "I hire good people, and I expect them to do their job. I'm here to support you, but it's your business." So you come in—you put your feet on the ground, and you're free.

Can I tell this story? I'm not on staff here. A couple nurses from the organization I work for had been in this facility previously. For whatever reason, it wasn't a good fit, and they were asked not to return. So when I went in my colleagues said, "You're going to Cathedral? Don't worry. You'll get kicked out. Everyone does." So I was terrified. I was waiting to get kicked out, and that never happened.

You know what? I figured something out. It wasn't Cathedral. It was the other nurses who had come to this facility. A nurse from the foundation told me, "We really like you because you care about these patients, and we can tell." That told me right there that's what they were looking for, and that's what they weren't seeing in my colleagues.

Now, when I walk in, I am treated like staff. I am treated like part of the family. So I can only imagine what it's like to really be in the whole scope of everything. They give you the opportunity to be in, but if you don't play fair, then you are not welcome. It's a close-knit group. They are very fair, but they will only give you three strikes and you're out.

Get It Done

Working here is really rewarding. If we pass by one of the residents they might not know your name, but they know who to call on to do certain things. It can be something simple like finding a piece of clothing. It might not be your job, but if you can, you get it done. That's it. That makes the residents comfortable. They will say, "I know if I came to you that you would get it done." So that makes your day.

There's nothing that Cathedral won't do for an employee. The only thing you need to do is be honest about what you want and what you need. If you come to me and I feel like it's legit, 9 ½ times out of 10 it's a done deal. That makes you feel good.

At one point in time, we really didn't have enough staff to make anybody the manager. We used what we could get to get through the day. So we looked at that. I didn't do anything right off. We kind of named one person as the supervisor or the "person you go to," but with perseverance and coming to work every day, people began to see a little improvement.

I remember that the first year I was here on Christmas Eve another person and I worked. We had both worked all day, and we didn't have anybody to do the cart that evening. I said to my colleague, "Let's hit it." She was my right-hand lady. She jumped right in, and we passed medications. I remember very well Christmas Eve night we both could hardly walk, but there was still that pride. We did it. She and I patted each other on the back and said, "All right girl, we did it." That was the kind of attitude that the staff needed to see. The other nurses have started doing the same now. All of the nurses at the time were working gobs of hours because this is what we had to do to get it done.

In our building, the elevator is our primary source of getting anywhere or getting anything. When the elevator doesn't work, we have to look at how we are going to get our dietary trays upstairs. One day when the elevator didn't work, someone said, "Okay, we can do the water brigade." So I went to the basement and started the brigade. I thought, "How much fun we're having! I'm glad that someone thought of doing this." It was a way to get it done.

I think that the one thing that is foremost with me is honesty. I can take anything as long as you're honest with me. If you are not honest, there is no relationship for me. So when people say, "Are we going to get a raise?"

I tell them, "I don't know. I honestly do not know if we are going to get a raise, but I know we are working on the budget." So I try to be as honest with them as I can. I'll say, "I'll tell you what. I will not take a raise until you get a raise. I'm going to bat for you. I've got a job to do, and I'm going to get it done."

I'm responsible and accountable for taking care of the residents, taking care of my staff, and helping out with other nurses. For me, I really don't consider myself above the other nurses. We are equal. What I preach I do. I usually come here early so that I can get things done. Not a day passes that my staff doesn't say, "Come help me with this." They tell me, "It's different when you're around. When you are around everything is done." When they need something, I will provide it for them right away. If I have to do a CNA job, I will. What satisfies them is that we help each other. The CNAs hug me because they know that I help and not just give orders.

Cathedral is the epitome of empowerment. We run our own little business, basically. We have all of the support we need. Autonomy is a good phrase for that, but we are all interconnected. We are totally 100% empowered to do what we need to do to get the job done—all of the way from the CEO to the staff. My expectation of my staff is for them to do their job without me having to hover over them. So they take ownership of their area. That's one of the things that really impressed me about this organization. It's hard to believe that there is such an organization, but there is—this is it.

When the administrator offered me the DON position, she asked me what would it take to get me to come work here. I said, "There were a few things that I insist that you do before I make that step: number one, that we would have supplies; number two that I would have a free reign in hiring and firing; and number three, let me alone and let me set it up. You can judge it from the actions."

"That is not a problem. You will have supplies; you will have money to do what you need to do." Since that time I've had a great relationship with her. She is my chief executive officer. She has given me free reign to do almost anything I wanted to do; she has been 100% supportive. She lets us grow. She is not a micromanager. She savors the good things that go on here.

Every nursing home has a survey each year. When the survey team is done, we sit down as a group, and we look at what we got tagged for. We ask ourselves, "What can we do to make this better next year?" The whole group participates. They know we have to look at the situation. Whether it was salt left on a tray or somebody gasping for breath, it's the same principle. We've had to fix it, and get it done well.

Positive Focus

I am here to have a positive impact on the role of the residents, the staff, and the family members. Also, I need to see where we are going in the future and not stay complacent. We need to see the opportunities ahead of us and change the involvement in the lives of the residents. We want to see growth for the residents as individuals and the family members, too.

I tell my staff to look at the positive—don't look at the negative. There will always be negatives in your life. You focus on the positives, and you'll come out with a smile.

The way I see it is if you want to do your job and you do your best, you will get the most out of it. If you come with a negative attitude, that's the attitude you will have all day. I came from a poor family, and my grandmother, mother, and father always instilled in me, "Hey, you help somebody, and that's where your blessings and rewards come from."

You are always going to have negative people. What I do with negative people is treat them nice. I do anything that I can do for them, and I then say, "God bless them" and move on.

A lot of times I wake up and come to work thinking, "If I can just get to work, something is going to happen that will get me through. Someone will say something to me or give me a little bit of wisdom or a little bit of love, and it will be just enough to get me through the next hour." Then someone else will say something. The next thing I know my day is gone, and I'm completely covered. Everything I need I can probably get here. I just like coming here.

She always encourages us to be happy and to be fulfilled whatever you're doing. She calls it the toxic thing. You don't want to be somewhere where you are picking up toxic, negative things. Here they encourage you. I can go somewhere and make more money, but would it be fulfilling like this place? Would they support me? Would they encourage me? Here they encourage you to be more than you can be. I like being here because my administrator and department heads are different from any other jobs I've had. They are not sticky and stuck-up.

Seeing employees that have changed has been the greatest thing. They continue to want to be involved here and to better their future by going back to school, or whatever it takes, to further themselves. A lot of the staff members are in the roles they are in because of their limitations. Many of them weren't blessed with families like myself. These people don't have that same encouragement, motivation, and lifestyle that I have. So, I try to get them on the right track and then keep them on the right track. I try to get people to believe in themselves and not just to be a "yes man" to others. I want them to know that within themselves they can make a change and a difference. When I look at where they were and where they've come to and hear them motivate others to do the same. It is rewarding.

Believing in People

The key element in a leader is to develop those good qualities and understate those bad qualities. If you are able to do that, then you get the best people can offer. Ultimately, you will reach your goals. I remember one of our people here. She worked with me in a different facility. In that other facility, there were some issues that were recognized, and they were putting her down. They were not taking advantage of what she had to offer. They were honing in on all of the negatives that that person had. Well, that particular person came to this building and applied for a job. I was asked if we should hire that person. I said, "Yes, let's go ahead because everyone has certain qualities that certainly we might be able to develop." The person was hired and has evolved and became a key person in the organization. My position was to reinforce the good elements that she brought in. That encouraged her to do better.

We have a physician assistant who works here. In my mind, she is a very compassionate, very involved, and very good provider. In a different facility, those attributes were her undoing. Even though that particular facility was a profitable one for our corporation, we pulled out of our business with them. That demonstrated how much we appreciated what she has done here. Those attributes, the positive attributes that I mentioned, were ones that she practices on a day-in and day-out basis. There's hardly a week that passes that I don't give her a call just telling her how much I appreciate what she does. Beyond that, at different times in the course of the year, I send gifts or flowers, all in appreciation of what she contributes to the residents here.

You can always get to where you need to be if you approach it in the proper manner and if you approach it in increments. Sometimes you want to throw so much stuff at people—it can be negative. Any negative you project will give you negatives in return, but if you project positives, people are going to respond positively.

One of my managers was in his first management role. He was frustrated with an employee who didn't do what she had been told. He wanted to fire her. I told him, "Step back and cool off. Look at all of the good things she does and talk to her about it. Give her some counseling. Don't be so fast to want to fire her. Everybody does things differently, and nobody is going to do things perfect all of the time."

The backbone of any facility is the CNAs. They can either make or break you in long-term care. Our director of nursing has a relationship with her CNAs that I have never witnessed in any other facility. They look at her as being their mother, their grandmother, their sister, their financial advisor, and their provider. She is the backbone to those CNAs. She can call one of them in and talk to them and help them to move and do the things that no other person will probably be able to. It's amazing. She treats them like those are her babies, but they work and they have a relationship. It's amazing.

We have CNAs who have gone on to further their education. That is a big stepping stone for the folks here because so many feel like they would never do any better. This was their life, and here we go. Several of them have gone ahead and done scholarships and have taken the GED and have furthered their education. I have several that are working for me now in a position as an LPN, and I consider us very fortunate. I enjoy seeing them grow. I see them getting out of that mold because this is the heart of Jacksonville. These girls have the ability to further their education and to do something for themselves.

One CNA really wanted to go to school, but she didn't think she could. She wanted to try. I said, "This is the thing. If you try, even if you fail, you can come back. So let's try it. I'll work with you. I'll send you to school, and I'll pay your tuition. I'll work with your schedule when you have to be in school. We can make this so that you can work weekends, and you can still support your family."

She passed her boards, and she now works for us as an LPN. She's absolutely wonderful. She has great leadership abilities and is a very fine nurse. We also had with us a gentleman who we supported through LPN school. Now he is one of the finest nurses we have.

We have yearly evaluations. When I, as the head nurse, make my evaluations, I evaluate my staff objectively. I say, "These are your weaknesses, and these are your strengths. You have potential. You can be a very good nurse or CNA. You can be a leader who influences other CNAs." When I do that, they change their ways for the better.

When I first got here I was going through a transition, and my manager was absolutely the most wonderful man I have ever met. He was always genuinely concerned, and he was always there for me. At the time, I was going through something. I was taking medication, and I was just a total wreck. He would always ask me, "How much can you handle? What can you do? What can we do to assist you?" Many times I would come in here, and I wouldn't have the words to say it. He would just help me through. He would help me to understand that I was going to have difficult days and that a lot of things are not fair. He was just always there.

The Unexpected

I am not a staff member, but I love coming here. I'll go up to the floor to see patients, and the staff will be singing and dancing and interacting with the patients. The next thing I know I'm singing and dancing and interacting with the patients. I feel like I belong here.

We are all expected to be professional. We are all expected to do our job. We are all expected to endure the stress. We are all expected to perform and to be responsible and accountable. We know that coming into our jobs. That's an expectation anywhere. Here, I feel it's about the unexpected.

You don't expect that open door policy where you can say anything to pull together and resolve an issue. You don't expect that personal attention outside of the job and the extra mile that administration goes. You don't expect that reaching out. Even though we all have our moments, we stand together. I think that's an important. It's what's expected here. It fosters our feelings and feeds our emotions.

If you have a problem and you take it to administration, they are more than happy to help you out. For instance, one person is going through some personal problems right now, and the foundation is splitting half the bills. You can't think of many companies that would do that for him. Plus, I would cry if he leaves.

One of the big headaches of the environmental services director anywhere is turnover. I had one person leave in two years, and he died. He couldn't help it, and we didn't kill him, by the way.

The thing that this job has that other jobs do not have is that they provide a safety net for their employees at all levels. No one is perfect 100% of the time, and you always have that someone that will reach out and take you in, hug you, and help you achieve some resolution.

We talk about the caring core of the administration and the staff at the Cathedral. Approximately five years ago we had a young lady who came to us to work as a CNA. She was 18 years old, her first job, from Haiti, away from her parents and her immediate family. A couple years after this young lady came to work with us, she became totally disabled. Last week this young lady came back into our facility, and the sole reason for coming was to talk to someone about her health and her personal needs. She had been gone approximately three years, very, very sick, and she came back to Cathedral. We were blessed to have her come back to nursing because she was one of ours, but she came back for that support that she knew that she could get it here, even though she no longer worked here. They know that when they leave that they can return, that we will be here. We did our best to set her up with some programs and some community support systems. In a nutshell that's who we are. That's what we do.

We have an employee that worked with us in the dietary department. She didn't have enough money to get her medication. She was sitting with her head on the table, and the CEO came up and asked what was wrong. She said, "I didn't get my medication. I didn't have enough money to get it." The CEO said, "Put 90 day's worth of her high blood pressure medicine on the nursing home credit card, and let's find access to medications for her." So it was like that.

We had a resident who expired yesterday. The resident's family member was here afterward and said, "You know I'm not staying away." He was connected to us and wanted to remain a part of this family.

I said to him, "Well you know we have a volunteer package for you with an assigned set of duties for you." He was laughing with us as he was packing up his mother's personal belongings. It was truly amazing. People come back. Cathedral is different. We are a different type of facility.

I've been affiliated with Cathedral for just over a year now. Often we have home patients that need placement. I recommend Cathedral every time. There's no comparison hands down. The patient care is—I just can't even describe it. The patient care is remarkable. These people that work here they love these patients. This is their mom and their dad. You don't see that everywhere.

I don't see the turnover here. For the year that I've been coming here, I have dealt with almost the same people on a daily basis. At any other nursing home, the turnover is daily. You are lucky to see the same person that you saw two days before. That goes from the housekeeping up to the top. So that tells me something is going on. They feel good about coming here for whatever reasons.

I have never seen a patient in Cathedral with significant skin breakdown. It doesn't happen because skin issues are addressed immediately and resolved. You will not see that anywhere else.

We all go to the CEO's house. It's not just the management level it is CNAs, housekeepers, and the dietary aides all mixed in together. We got to know each other more and learn a little bit more about each other as individuals. To me that says a lot for our CEO. How many CEOs are going to invite their hourly people into their home, feed them, and offer them all the hospitality in the world? It just doesn't happen.

We are not just people who work together. We are family. When you wake your boss up at 2:00 in the morning and she is sweet enough to say, "What can I do for you? What do you want me to do to help?" To me that says that I'm not just your boss. I'm your friend, and I will do for you whatever I can to help.

Respecting Diversity

You are not going to change these folks. You accept them for what they are.

The Cathedral Foundation is inclusive and eclectic. Years ago I had a little cartoon about how an organization, if its board chairman is wearing a bowtie, then all of the other people on the board are wearing bow ties. That certainly couldn't be said about Cathedral. There's every walk of life, every color, and every set of life experiences. Instead of trying to homogenize all of that, somehow we can work with uplifting all of that as part of who we are.

One employee came, and she was in a panic because she had lost her daughter. This was the day that she was getting her daughter back. They had taken her for a while. She had no idea what was going to happen. She had no food in the house and no bus fare. She was said, "I don't know what to do. They are going to drop her off right now. Can you help?" I made a few phone calls to the foundation, and they gave her money to buy food, transportation, and everything for her and her child. This building, this company, reaches out to the employees personally. It's really nice working here.

I am not from America originally. I'm from Sudan. I left my country because the civil war tore the country apart. I came here looking to get an education. Cathedral is helping me to get my CNA license, and now I got my GED diploma.

As a whole, people enjoy coming to work here. I think we all like to do a good job. We like to laugh and kid and joke. We know what we need to do and when we need to do it. I think a lot of times the staff are friends and not just co-workers. They care about each other as individuals. They are supportive of each other and their family needs in a crisis.

I had been unemployed for about four years. I have a son who has autism, so he's in a group home. I just got up one day and put in an application. I had never worked in a nursing home before but I needed a job. Cathedral called and offered me a job. It was very nice. First, I was a little timid because it was something new to me, but I liked the people in management. Everybody was just eager to work with me on situations and help me. It's been seven years now, but they still ask, "Are you okay? What can we do to help you?" It is always a family atmosphere. They will work with you, work around your time, and adjust time. It has always been that way. It's not just my department. It's everywhere.

What keeps me at Cathedral is that I've grown and matured working here. I've learned different things about myself, and I've learned it from my job. When I first got here I was just getting out of rehab, and they were supportive of my meetings. I could go and talk with them when I'm having real bad days. Some days I have even asked, "You know I really need to get to a meeting today." I was transitioning from a different time where I was coming into the working class and doing what working people do: pay bills and work.

Now, I have a different insight toward life. I have learned communication skills by dealing with the residents. I've learned about acceptance, patience, and teamwork. I take a lot of these tools home and use them with my family and friends. They just took my hand and helped me grow.

Cathedral has affected me spiritually. I stopped here one day because it was hot out and it was air conditioned. I was going to sit here to cool off and collect the job application. The receptionist encouraged me to fill out the application, and then said she'd put a star by my name. When I asked her why, she said, "I don't know, but something told me to put a star by your name." The receptionist could tell I really needed the job. Within a week I got the job. So I don't call that a coincidence. I call that "God gave me a gift."

There is never a problem if you have some kind of issue. You can talk with someone, and they will do whatever they can do to assist you. When my schooling came up, I just gave them a schedule of what days I go to school, and then we adjusted my schedule. We just went from there. It was never an issue.

I have a nurse manager, and she is probably one of the finest young nurses that I've ever worked with. She had to get certified here, so we got that done. She was well mannered and very soft spoken and had difficulty being direct. Initially, I had to take care of all her disciplinary actions. She would come to me and say, "I can't do this."

I placed her in a position on the floor where my office is. I figured that I could kind of watch what was going on. I would tell her, "You don't know how well you are doing! You are going to get a little tougher skin. You are going to get out there, and you are going to do it." Now she is quite successful as a manager.

I had one nurse; she was a little girl who had no training. She said she would like to try it. She was good with charting, and so we trained her. I sent her to Ostomy school down in Fort Lauderdale, and she got her certification. She's been with me ever since and has done really a remarkable job.

We had a resident who had come from the Salvation Army. When it was time to discharge her, everybody was all in a dither. We have no place to send her. We asked her where she would go after she left here. She said, "Well I'm going back to the Salvation Army—$10.00 a night, best place I've ever been." So we took her to get her Social Security check and then to the bank, and she returned to the Salvation Army. I don't care what we would have done for her. Even if we put her in the Taj Mahal, she would have gone back to the Salvation Army. That's her choice. We are not going to change it.

Elder Angels

I am the coordinator for the fire department, and we do different things for different people. The Elder Angels program started when we received a call from a lady that was a friend of a resident. She called our volunteer person and asked if we could help buy a Cathedral resident a dress to wear to church. At the time, we had already adopted another agency to donate to. We told her that at this time we really didn't have anything. Still, she gave us the lady's sizes and everything.

Well, we sent all of our gifts to our other program, and there was an extra gift left over. When we opened it, we saw that it was exactly the Cathedral resident's size, and it was almost exactly the dress that the lady wanted.

So we brought it down to Cathedral, and the lady was so excited. She said, "That is exactly what I wanted." She just couldn't believe it. She had kind of given up on going to church that day. It was like a blessing. It was like an angel somewhere.

The Jax Care Program is a city team of volunteers. Since the lady-with-the-dress incident, we adopt Cathedral residents that don't have any family, and we provide Christmas for them. We volunteer our time to go out and buy things that they need. It's kind of a special little deal between them and us. It's really exciting.

When we first started this program quite a few years ago, my son and I would bring the gifts down on Christmas Eve. Personally, I don't have any grandparents living, so it's kind of exciting to come here and see them. My son just enjoys hearing the stories that the people tell, so it has kind of helped him like the elderly and grow as a person. He is going into the medical field because of this.

The staff members are so appreciative. They are really excited about the program. They wait for us to call every year to see if we are going to adopt. They say, "Oh, you are all coming back this year?"

I'll say, "You got me a list?"

They say, "We were waiting on you all."

The last couple of years that we came in with vans full of Christmas gifts. The residents are waiting. There may be two out there at first and then in a little while there's like 20. Many come rolling down. They come from nowhere. They say, "Did you bring me something? Did you bring me something?"

We take gifts upstairs to the bedridden ones, and they are really excited to see someone come visit them and talk to them. There's one man up there who every year asks for chewing tobacco. He's really old, and so usually that's the one my son and I adopt. He always wants a baseball cap from some team, and he always wants something really neat. So we kind of sneak him in a little tobacco. What's it going to hurt? He always sees us coming, and he knows he's going to get something good. He can't get out of bed so he just sits up and puts his hat on. He gets really excited.

Cathedral serves a lunch for the volunteer people. The guests come in and they have a few of the residents sit down there with us. We sit at tables. We talk to them, and they tell us some of the stories of their old times, which is kind of neat. There is a fire station across the street, and after 9/11, we had a luncheon for them. After that, we just got close with them and the people at the city office. Sometimes we call and invite the fire department for a cook-out. The residents come and sit and talk to us, and we mingle with them. It's really cool.

There was this one lady here who never came out of her room at all. She had seen these buff guys from the fire department coming in here all dressed up. So she got all dressed up and came to the lunch. She rolled over in her wheel-chair and was feeling some of the guys' muscles. They became friends with her. In fact, she went upstairs and got some dollar bills—it was so funny—and rolled her wheelchair right down there, and she was wondering who was going to dance! She said that some of them looked like her husband. They became friends with her and they started coming over here and visiting her. They take her across the street over to the fire department to eat lunch and show her around. Every year they adopted her until she passed. So that was kind of exciting.

My grandparents passed away—all four of them when I was very young. So I never had the opportunity to get to know them. Thus, I guess I just kind of adopt all of the residents. They are like my grandmothers and grandfathers. I try to do everything I can to make their life as pleasant as possible. If they have an idea, if they want to do it, and if it's doable, I do it.

It makes us feel like we've really done something for the citizens. They've helped us over the years, and now it's our turn to help them.

Near as Home

There's one thing I must say. Near as home this place is.

They are very good, very nice. Most all of them who wait on me are very nice.

I came out here and I got along real good. I get along with the nurses and get along with the CNAs, and I don't want to go home now. It's 'bout closest to home as you can get.

Well, they treat me as an individual. They treat me real nice, and I treat them real nice. So it comes back to you.

It can't get lonesome for activities. They have all kinds here. They take us shopping, and we come back all laden down with the things we bought. We are happy.

We even went on a cruise last year. We really enjoyed it. Everybody was so nice. They had the girls who work here to go with us and assist with anything we wanted. My caretaker went with me and carried me because I don't get around very much.

They have cabs out to lunch, cabs to go shopping at least once a month, and then they have Bingo. They have church service here, real good church service.

I've been to other homes, and I've never seen so many activities. They even have a doggy day where people can bring their pets in. I happened to come last time during Bingo, and half of the residents weren't in their rooms because they were at Bingo. When they came back from Bingo, they all had glowing faces. This place is awesome.

The food and everything here is good. They make the best soup in Jacksonville. My mom thinks I come to visit her just to eat.

They have some good down-home cooking.

We have ice cream every Sunday.

Tuesday is tea day, ladies tea.

Once a month we have a candlelight dinner. The residents choose their menu, and sometimes it's really wild. Dietary prepares it. The department heads, and other people serve it. They have had everything from steak to shrimp. The residents really look forward to it.

If a resident has lost her daughter or their son, the staff is there for them, to be their friend, to sit there and hold their hand, let them talk about their problems. If it's their birthday and they have no family, people take up money and go get them a birthday gift or cards or send them a balloon. They get them a Kentucky Fried Chicken meal or go across the street to Winn Dixie and get their favorite foods. They let them use their cell phone to call a brother or sister. They bring them clothes from home, buy them brand new clothes, or bring stuff for their grandchild.

If one person can't get what the resident needs, they will tell others and collect the money they need. There is always willingness to work together to get the task accomplished. Then you don't hear about it from the staff person who took the collection. You hear it from somebody else—an observer. So they aren't doing it for show. They do it to provide residents what they need.

They go to see the resident while they are away in the hospital because they miss them and miss talking to them. They spend time with a family member because they need that encouragement. I think seeing that they care is shown throughout the facility at all levels.

I don't think you could find a better place. I know some that cost a lot more money, but they are no better. You can spray paint anything over, but it don't make it better.

It's been real nice, and I don't have any complaints. If I see anything that needs to be done, they go ahead and do it. Very seldom do I have to ask them to do anything. So I'm real glad of that. The atmosphere is real nice.

When I first came here I said, "Now this is the place for me." I'm really blessed to be put in a place like this, and I really take my hat off to the nurses and to the staff. They have been very cooperative with me because if I ask them for something, they go and do it. If I say that I don't like that thing, they will ask me if I want something else. I find it very nice, really nice.

I had been suffering for quite some time with my feet swelling. When I came here for rehab I said, "You know—I don't have anybody to take care of me. I'm going to ask them, 'Can I be a resident and patient?'" The very next day I asked, and they told me that I could if that's what I wanted. I needed to be some place that they can see about me and see what I need. I'm very satisfied.

My sister is here. When she came here, she said, "Let me stay there for a while and see what it's like." She came and stayed. She said, "You know it's kind of nice here to have somebody waiting on you, getting you food three times a day and snacks, and everybody is so nice. They treat me so nice. I get cold at night, but when I tell them I'm cold, they give me more covers to put on the bed. The nurses, the workers, the kitchen help, everybody—they are very nice." I would recommend it any day.

It would seem like I would worry about her, but I don't because I know where she's at. I know they are taking care of her, and I'm not talking about who's in charge of the place. I'm talking of people who lay on the floor, go down there, take care of her, wake her up to go eat, and hug her. Folks here are her family now. You can cut it anyway you want to, but that's the way it boils down to.

This is as close to home as we are going to get.

Editor Commentary

It's most unusual to have a "nonmission" statement, especially in an organization so clearly mission driven as Cathedral, but this unique approach is clearly a defining aspect of the organization. Connecting each individual employee's core purpose, gifts, and talents to achieving the organization's goals, every day, is where the magic happens.

Senior leadership articulated a "different vision" of aging and was brave enough to recognize that "how it has always been done" wouldn't work for them; thus, it would need to be changed—beginning with them. That new vision drives the entire organization, and it makes its way to individual encounters between residents and employees every day.

All of this is accomplished with and through an abiding and embedded love for their residents as individual people with lives and goals. They accept them, encourage them, care for them, and care about them at whatever level of individual physical and mental capabilities. The involvement of the residents in the community and of community members with the residents is creative and unusual in many long-term care settings. The stories from the community members are particularly poignant.

The highly visible leadership at the nursing home—the CEO and the CNO especially—are particular standouts in this regard; they set the standards for excellence every day. Their role modeling is extraordinary. The respect they have for their employees, and the underlying confidence that they have in them shines through. The employees clearly articulate what a difference this makes to them and how that translates into their ability to make a difference for the residents. Certified nursing aides (CNAs) practically live with the residents, and they become family to each other. The nurses, aides, and support staff at Cathedral exhibit a high level of teamwork and trust in each other. Ongoing coaching and teaching, especially through the use of storytelling, occur throughout the organization.

The care that leaders take in selecting the right employees is apparent in several stories. Although it might seem expedient to take "the next warm body," the leaders are committed to making sure that they have the right person for the job. Their commitment to developing human potential even extends to those applicants that they don't hire by letting them know they will be successful somewhere else, even if they aren't a good fit for this position.

Human potential—whether that of the resident or the employee—is valued, developed, and encouraged throughout Cathedral. The leaders provide the support that employees need to be successful in their current jobs and are given the confidence to learn and grow in their personal and professional lives.

Table 10-1   Organizational Demographics

Organization	Greenwich Hospital, a member of the Yale New Haven Health System
Location	Greenwich, CT
Setting	Suburban
Communities served	Suburban
Type of organization	Greenwich Hospital is a not-for-profit community teaching hospital.
Number of beds	174
Number of FTEs	1,484
Scope of service	Greenwich Hospital is a full-range community teaching hospital offering medical, surgical, diagnostic, and preventative services.
Organizational awards	In Fiscal Year 2006, Greenwich Hospital was recognized for the high quality of care provided by the Hospital. Governor Rell came to Greenwich Hospital to conduct a public signing of a state health care law. Governor Rell signed the act at Greenwich Hospital due to the hospital's excellent low infection rates and cited it as an institution providing the highest quality of care.
	2006 Silver Connecticut Quality Improvement Award
	Partnership's CQIA Innovation Prize for its results on the prevention of central venous catheter-related blood stream infections.
	Primary Stroke Center
	Sleep laboratory was upgraded to sleep center status by the American Academy of Sleep Medicine
	"Top 100 Most Wired Hospitals" by *Hospitals and Health Networks* magazine for the sixth year in a row
	Center for excellence in geriatric care, a national award given by the AGS. The emergency department nursing staff was named among the "Best Nursing Teams for 2006" by ADVANCE *for Nurses* newsmagazine for "adaptability and initiative" relating to increased patient demand and new programs for stroke and heart attack. Greenwich Hospital continued to excel in patient satisfaction measures and for the past 22 consecutive quarters has been ranked in the top percentiles of all hospitals in the nation (as measured by Press Ganey); 2 quarters at the 98th percentile and 20 quarters at the 99th percentile.
Focus area	Inpatient medical care units, including general medicine and medical oncology
Focus area served	In FY 2005, these departments had a total of 3,015 inpatient discharges.
Focus area best practices and awards	Individual staff members in the focus area have been recognized by patients and colleagues through the monthly quality award program at Greenwich Hospital.
	Greenwich Hospital's Medical Oncology unit has increased patient satisfaction from a low of the 70th percentile in December of 2004 to the 99th percentile as of June 2006. The overall rating of care was scored by patients as 97.4.
	Agency staff is not used in any of the medical areas included in the focus group. Staff turnover remains below the national average.

CHAPTER 10

Establishing Trust Through Consistency

Contributor: Carol Gorelick

The stories in this chapter are the voices of the Greenwich Hospital CEO, the COO, the vice-president of patient and guest relations, the service excellence steering committee, two patient care directors, a nurse manager, staff from the medical oncology unit, and their patients. Here are their stories.

GREENWICH HOSPITAL: A MEMBER OF THE YALE NEW HAVEN HEALTH SYSTEM

Service Journey

Back in 1998 or 1999, I actually chaired meetings with every employee in the institution. We met around the clock. I must have had 30 to 40 meetings. Every employee had to go. During that meeting, I told them about the service journey we were going to take and how we were going to change the culture of this organization to one that was really obsessed with quality and service. We wanted every employee to come on that journey with us.

One of the first things that we did was focus on getting our whole organization tied together in terms of what we call the MVVG—Mission, Vision, Values, and Goals. We asked every department to create a team to do their own values statements and goals. We had more than 600 people involved in that process. At the conclusion of the Mission, Vision, Values, and Goals activity, we asked all of the departments to put together a poster presentation of their department's goals. We had a big event called Mission–Vision–Values–Goals Day. It was a festive environment with popcorn and balloons. There were probably 50 or 60 posters around the room. We asked somebody from every department to explain them. We invited all of the employees down to the auditorium to come and see these. It was amazing to see the presentations and the creativity. There was just a whole level of enthusiasm and excitement.

We had employees develop some service standards. I didn't want the standards to come from me. So we took the Employee of the Year winners from the past 10 or 11 years, got them together, and said, "All right, you guys are the leaders of Greenwich Hospital. What service standards should we have?" They came up with our seven service standards. We overhauled the performance appraisal system, and those standards were literally written right into the performance appraisal.

   Then we had every employee sign off on these standards. We then said, "Okay, we've got to walk the talk." Let's make a 60% merit increase for employees based on how their manager feels they are meeting those standards. Each year we set patient satisfaction score targets and financial targets, and if we hit those targets, every single employee has additional money put into a retirement plan. The longer you've been here, the greater the percentage. So it's also a retention tool. The last three years we have been able to pay out employee incentive, that extra piece that goes into the retirement plan.

At every leadership meeting we talk about patient satisfaction, and one of the things I want to make sure of is, because we are so high, that we don't get complacent. At every single leadership meeting, I try and find a way to get people re-motivated. The meetings are monthly, and patient satisfactions are a daily game. It's an hourly game, and you can't lose any of those games if you want to stay on top. So my thought process was that here we have a move coming up. We are going to be talking about patient satisfaction, and let's see if we can challenge the group to step up to the plate and not only have the move go without a hitch; however, let's see if we can come through a move and kind of break trend (that is, have our scores stay steady during that period of time), and they did pretty much.

There was a particular leadership meeting where I felt that we were coasting in terms of people's effort with regard to patient satisfaction. I asked myself how I was going to handle it. Was I going to be angry, or was I going to try to motivate people? I decided to go the route of motivation, which is always the right way. I talked a little bit about what our vision was and what we had built here over the past 10 to 15 to 20 years. I took them back to what this hospital was like back then. The before and after is just unbelievable; it's kind of like, if you see it, it's just two different organizations. I asked them if they were satisfied with mediocrity.

I reminded them that when we hired them they signed on to an organization that was progressive, cared about patients, and would never stop raising the bar. I told them that to some degree I was disappointed. I felt that people were not challenging their staff and were not motivating their staff to raise the bar. I did not want to become a mediocre organization. Even though our scores were high, we needed to constantly push to raise the bar. They needed to decide whether or not they wanted to be part of something great or just something good. My hope was that they would be part of something great.

I asked for suggestions. It started off slowly. People came up with suggestions, and I could see that they were engaged. They were going to do what they could to raise the patient satisfaction scores. I believe that as soon as you take your foot off the gas you lose the edge when it comes to that kind of culture. You can't allow even three or four employees to talk negatively about people. You can't stand for that. I put a lot of pressure on people to constantly stay at that level.

I felt after that meeting that people were re-energized and knew what our mission was and knew where we wanted to go and where we wanted to be. I think they were embarrassed to some degree because they hadn't been pushing. I got feedback from people about that. So I felt that that particular meeting was a very, very positive experience.

We establish goals every year. We have fiscal goals. We have patient satisfaction goals. They are all components of whether or not, if we meet those goals, we receive an additional incentive bonus. With nonexempt employees, they typically receive money into their annuity funds. With exempt employees, it is actually a cash bonus. So every employee knows. We are very, very heavily weighted, and a component of that incentive is our patient satisfaction scores. We set certainly not levelized, but achievable goals, and everyone in the institution knows that we need to make them across the board. So, every person is a player in that patient satisfaction scorecard, and if we achieve those goals, it's a little bit of extra money in our pocket. If we don't, we strive harder the next year. So far, we've been very lucky that we have been able to achieve them, but everyone knows it's not a given.

I don't think the incentive bonuses are really the driver for service excellence. I think they are more of recognition. The typical employee here is driven by where we are, what the goals are, and to be the best we possibly can.

It's not whether we achieve. Those numbers are set by administration and are benchmarks for us to achieve, but I don't think any of us are looking at the numbers saying, "Oh, we are two points below this. I'm not going to get my bonus." It just doesn't work that way.

The Essence of Leadership

I am not the leader. My people lead me and make me who I am. If I don't have good staff, there's no way I am going to be able to lead them. So, it needs to start right down with the lay staff. If you can build a trusting relationship with them, it will work. I think there are very trusting relationships right from the CEO through the COO, through the program directors, and on to the staff.

I admire my manager. He speaks clearly about the values that have driven our success. When he wants us to work hard. We see him working hard. When he tells us to be responsive, we see him clearly setting the standard. He believes in us and we believe in him.

At a meeting one person stood up and said, "Maybe you should think about coming to all of our departmental meetings to motivate the staff." I said I would be happy to come to the departmental meetings, but it's your job to motivate the staff. It's the manager and supervisor's job. You are the leaders in your unit. We don't want people to respond to the CEO applying pressure. We want it to be part of the culture, and you can instill culture in your work unit. That's your job, and everybody was kind of like, "Yeah. Wow. That's true." That was a defining moment.

Every Wednesday's leadership meeting contains patient satisfaction updates. The service excellence committee is about 35 to 40 managers, and together we go through the entire report. The expectation is that managers will have gone through the complaints, researched them, and will be prepared to talk about how we can take the complaint "off the radar screen." That has had a dramatic effect in bringing our organization together to focus on service excellence. There isn't a meeting that we don't talk about service excellence. It is part of everything that we do.

The goal of the meetings is to help others with their service excellence. During these meetings, the CEO and I sit across from each other at the table so that I can read him and he can read me. I watch his delivery, and I try to pay attention to him; however, I'm also looking and listening to others. What I really want to do is look around the table to see how people are hearing the news. I want to see which person it is bothering the most and what type of follow-up I might do with that person. I was trying to listen to the nurse manager next to me, but she was very quiet. I heard a couple of surprised gasps at the other end of the table from directors. I was thinking that I needed to come back to them after the meeting. I think people did okay with the news.

What I appreciate in working with our CEO is that he's decisive. You can talk with him about something. He will quickly make a decision, and he will stand by it.

Our nurse manager sets the tone for our staff. She is the first to make the department customer friendly for patients and staff. She will work seven days a week if we don't have ideal coverage. She covered for one nurse in the emergency department during one annual holiday party so that the nurse could attend the party. She walks the walk regarding service.

The CEO, COO, and administration, they are not untouchable. They are out here among the people. They walk through. They know our names. They know the housekeepers, and everybody has input. Your opinion is valued whether you are a housekeeper, a nurse, an aide, or a physician. They listen to you. Not that they fix everything the way I want it or the way you want it, but your voice is heard. They reward people for service excellence on a monthly basis, and so, if you saw a good deed or you heard a good story, they have a tea and read the stories out loud. We applaud our comrades because the work that gets done here is amazing.

Our clinical leader teaches service excellence to the staff and lives it every day. She makes rounds to all patients every day and works quickly to fix any problems they may have. Many of our patients comment on patient satisfaction surveys that the clinical leader fixed their problems for them. She is well liked and respected by the staff.

I'm the type of individual who will make myself as visible as I can. I get to work at 7:00 a.m., and I walk through all my areas of responsibility. I take a quick walk through the building in about 30 minutes. I like to see the night staff going off so that they can share with me. I find it very pleasing to say "good morning!" to the people here at that time of the morning.

Here I feel like you are on your own departmental level. I'm free to make the decision that I need to make to get it done. Everybody on the team knows what needs to be done to get it done, and they get it done in an excellent kind of way.

You should always be ready for interruptions and be able to stop whatever you are doing at that moment to make time for whoever is coming into your office. Usually, whatever is on their mind is very important to them. They want an answer right then, or they want to be heard right then. You should be able to take the good with the bad because you get plenty of each.

Sometimes little things that are very inexpensive really go a long, long way. The closest thing to somebody's heart is how well you feed him or her. Going back as long as I can remember, I would go out and get a six-foot wedge, some sodas, and pizzas for my staff. Small things like that make a difference.

We are very short staffed at times, and when you're short staffed, it leads to a very stressful environment. The amount of support that I can provide the manager is critical. Radiology may have 30 or 40 cases, with 40 to 50 CAT scan patients to get done in an eight-hour period. In addition, the emergency department and inpatient are adding cases. There are patients sitting in the waiting room. This puts a lot of stress on the manager. One day, on top of all that, a piece of equipment went down. Now the manager is being pulled in many different directions. I had to get out on the floor and rub elbows with that manager, letting her know that I was there to help. So I think with that type of scenario I need to understand what the manager may need and deliver on it before being asked.

When my dad passed, the CEO of the hospital, the chief operating officer, and representatives of the entire administrative staff came to offer their condolences to my family. I don't live in town. I'm 60 miles from here.

Recognition comes in various forms of "pats on the back," but it's more. Superiors recognize not only your effort and your team's effort, but also the efforts of those family members who support you. When your VP sends flowers to your spouse, that really hits home. They recognize that we are working long hours and that things might be stressful at home because of it. That is a different type of recognition that is above and beyond and more personalized.

The Patient First

This is an organization that is driven by putting the patients first. I've worked in organizations where I've seen it be "just a job." I didn't go into nursing because I wanted to learn how to use a computer or how to be a business manager or just to do a job. Greenwich Hospital is a place where the patients are well taken care of and the team truly has a sense of caring. This is directly connected with my values. You can't compare this place with any other.

The vice president of patient and guest relations lives for patient satisfaction. She is a role model for the department as well as for the entire Greenwich Hospital community. One day our emergency department was overpacked, and she went into action. She gathered up people to help her move additional chairs into the hallway for the excess people to sit. She then met with all of the patients waiting and had conversations with them—making them feel at ease. On top of this, she was using a nearby phone to answer pages and make return phone calls—she is amazing!

We constantly do things here through the eyes of a patient, and everything we do is with the patient in mind. Whether it's an outpatient or an inpatient, it's all about those who we serve. If I didn't get any of these awards, I would be perfectly fine with it by just running into patients who say, "You know, you've got a great place here." That's enough of a reward for me.

Our staff really tries to take care of each patient as if they are the only one here. Each patient's care is the most important at the time. What stands out about these individuals is their commitment. They go out of their way to be helpful. They truly extend themselves.

We take care of the patient's needs in ways that are not medical, but are personal and psychological. Very simply, many people come to registration when they don't know where to go. The family member of a patient who was very ill was all alone one day. Three of my staff took it upon themselves to use their break and lunch time to keep the person company in her time of need and worry.

Before checking on a patient, I noticed it was her 92nd birthday, so I brought her some flowers with a happy birthday card. The guitar lady happened to be on that floor that day, so I asked if she would play happy birthday for the 92-year-old woman. It was great! The patient was very happy. A month later I was visiting one of our offsite facilities to do training with the staff, and a lady came up to me and says, "I just want to shake your hand and thank you for what you did for my mom last month." I was shocked. She explained that it was her mom who I gave the birthday flowers to. I turned red, but inside I felt so happy to have been able to touch someone's life in such a positive way. It really felt good, and I was honored to have experienced this.

It is better to know the patient who has a disease than to know the disease that has the patient. We see them as Mr. Brown with diabetes or Mrs. Smith with hypertension. So the focus really is on the individual rather than the disease process.

One particular patient had severe claustrophobia, and the lead MRI technician was not able to get the study done. The patient's exam was never completed, and thus, her visit was much shorter than anticipated. She had been dropped off at the hospital and now had no way of getting back home. The MRI technician felt responsible for the situation and took ownership of it. She comforted the patient, drove her home, and took her to her door.

The patient sent a nice letter to the CEO, and he cited it as an example at the service excellence meeting. We would have never known that the MRI technician did this if it weren't for the patient's letter. Further, it wasn't a clinical issue about a failed MRI. It was a "me as a person" issue. The patient said, "Look what Greenwich did for me."

Not every employee is going to jump in the car and take somebody home, but there are other things that employees do to alleviate high anxiety levels, stress levels, and concerns for our patients, and so, it's not a uniqueness, it's the culture.

We had to discharge a patient who didn't have any clothes. We called for clothes from the Greenwich auxiliary. The shoes they gave us were too small for the guy. I said, "Oh, my! It's 6:00 p.m., and the Auxiliary is closed." It became a team effort. A transport guy came. We thought everything was set. The patient was all dressed up, but he didn't have shoes. I couldn't discharge him without shoes. It was cold. The transport guy went home and got his new pair of shoes and gave them to the patient as well as a jacket. The patient—you could see his face—he was just so thankful. We gave him a taxi voucher and some extra food because it was a late discharge. That was something you don't forget.

We had a young woman who had a skiing accident and was going to be entering college in the fall. One of my orthopedic certified nurses took her under her wing. This young girl really wanted to have her hair washed or take a shower. Her friends were coming to visit, and they were going to be her roommates in college. We got the clearance. I was really impressed when the nurse walked in with her own bathing suit! The young woman was so nervous about standing with the instability of the fusion. So the nurse basically took a shower with the patient. Her mother was blown away. We couldn't stop the mother from crying. The young girl is getting ready to graduate from college this year, and she has maintained that personal tie with the nurse.

We had a patient who was in the hospital for a long period of time going through a treatment. What he really wanted was to see his animals. The staff didn't realize he had four really big dogs. The whole staff got together to try to sneak the dogs in. The dogs ran back and forth on the unit. The patient was having a great time. The dogs were so thrilled to see him. There was no control as the dogs ran around the rooms. The whole staff was involved in trying to get these animals upstairs. The bottom line is that if patients ask for things, it can be simple little things or bigger things. It seems that we have the ability to do what they ask for. It's not because it's an affluent hospital. If someone wants something, the whole team will get together, the whole hospital.

We had a patient who didn't tell anyone about her fear of an MRI until the exam was finished. Afterward, she told us it upset her because she was a 9/11 survivor. It bothered the tech so much all night that she just wanted to do something. The service recovery actually came from the staff member. It wasn't from the patient relations department. It came from the MRI tech. We sent her flowers, and the staff sent her flowers. It's so much better when you do it from the staff rather than from the organization or the department. It made for a personal connection.

It's not just the patient we take care of. We consider the families of our patients, too. There was a lady, a relatively young woman, who was with us for such a long period of time. Working with the husband and the daughter, it was so clear that, regardless of how much they knew about the woman's diagnosis, they weren't ready to let her go. I was listening and talking to the daughter and helping her to understand. She is 21 and an only child. The things she would say about her mother were just unbelievable. You get to really fall in love with the patient and the family. The daughter really touched me to the point where I had to go to her mother's wake to make sure that she was okay. She was so close to her mom. I read a poem she wrote about her mother. This is one of those things that I will remember forever.

A young woman who was not doing very well was given a very poor prognosis. It was her birthday. Knowing that it potentially could have been her last birthday, a staff nurse generated a trigger. He came up to me and said, "It's her birthday. Her kids are at school. What can we do?" I said to him, "We can do a lot." So I got on the phone and called our support person for guest relations. She went to the gift shop and bought a teddy bear. We called the dietary department, and I spoke to our director of dietary and asked him what we could possibly set up. "Can we do a mini birthday party after the kids got out of school, for mom and the kids, to celebrate her birthday?" He sent up a whole cookie tray with a cake and juices. I ran to Party City and picked up room decorations and balloons. We decorated her entire room. She was able to have a birthday celebration with her kids. She was extremely, extremely appreciative. There were family members who came as well as friends. It was just great! It probably took us all of about a half hour to pull the whole thing together. It just felt great. That's what we do on that unit.

One of the doctors told me that when you come here you don't receive special care because you are an employee; we give the same care across the board. I am an employee, and my son came in for an ear infection. The doctor wanted to do a 25-minute procedure. I was nervous because he's only two years old. I was an emotional wreck. So my wife took him to this procedure. All I can say is that my son, who is so fussy when it comes to absolutely everything, came home and said, "I had fun at the hospital."

My wife was actually in tears when she told me about the staff members who were dancing on their heads, bouncing up and down, and playing games with him. It just blew me away. The relief I felt because my son was so well taken care of and had a nontraumatic experience is huge. We register over 7,000 patients a week. Knowing that the majority of them are going home with the same type of relief is overwhelming.

Developing People

We encourage people to invest in themselves and their careers. The outcome is that they are able to provide a higher, more personal level of care than if we just dealt with the structure.

We've developed a mentoring program for new employees. The first couple of weeks for a new employee are the most essential in deciding if you like the place and the people and how well you are helped. We train long-term employees to be certified mentors who are assigned to new employees. They sort of shadow those employees during the first few weeks of the new position to help them with questions, show them the ropes, and get them through the hurdle of the new job experience.

I think the strongest thing you can do for an employee is to keep them educated and communicate to them, and we have a phenomenal education department here. With other facilities, I have found that when the money goes the first department to go is education. They cut conferences and education staff. I don't know what the mindset is behind that, to think it's okay. Do they think that the less educated staff we have the better we are going to be able to perform? It doesn't make sense, and I think we realize that here. We've invested heavily in a training program that every employee can take online to enhance his or her education. It's mandatory, absolutely, and it's part of the performance appraisal process: going through their mandatory sessions. It shows our commitment to investing in your staff and your own people. If you don't, there's no way you're going to make a superlative difference in how you treat your patients.

I think an extraordinary investment in people here is that the hospital is committed to provide a management course for leaders. I think to date there are 140 to 150 leaders in the organization who are graduates of the management course.

I looked at the opportunity to take the management course as a scholarship. I was only here for a few months when I was allowed to go to the class. It was amazing. This was just such an awesome opportunity to meet people in a different setting, build alliances with your peers, and learn an amazing skill set from the course.

We are wonderful at patient satisfaction. I have 30 minutes to explain the value of patient satisfaction scores to new folks in orientation. The way I teach is by telling stories and how to use feedback. I take our survey with me and teach the tool. First, I give them information and show them how we measure. I tell them what the results of the measure are. Then we talk about what we do with feedback. Once I go through the concrete details, I tell them a story. A patient was dying of leukemia, and his wife had just delivered their first baby. A nurse asked if we could install a web cam in the patient's home. We made it happen and gave this man and his wife a little unexpected joy.

By telling the story, the new employees understand that service excellence means always bumping up an idea. A staff member taking care of the patient can best assess the patient's need and ask the patient if implementing the idea would be useful. If the patient feels your idea would help, then you should ask, "What if?" Your goal should be to turn the idea into reality for the patient. When service excellence concepts are put into action, all of the pieces fall into place.

I was just in a class last night where somebody said, "Do you still tell that story?" That person actually repeated the short story that I had told them in their orientation class. I would never have known that people remember, but they identified with the story. That helped them to transition to doing great things in customer service.

It is an honor for me to watch nurses grow. We have taken several staff nurses in the oncology unit through the Student Internship Program. They developed and grew within the unit as staff nurses for two or three years. Then I worked with them to obtain their Oncology Nursing Certification through the Oncology Nursing Society. It really pushed them into being part of an affiliate organization. They are proud of their specialty. I guess the shining light for me is always to be part of the clinical career progression ladder. Each nurse has their own uniqueness and style, but the commonality is their commitment and dedication to the unit and to what they do on a day-to-day basis.

Many people come and go in their professions, and many don't have the level of commitment that this staff has. I think the mere fact that they stick with it is remarkable because oncology is a tough love. It is not something that everybody can do. To see them do it with passion and commitment and also mentor others just touches me deeply. To know that I can entrust them with patient care and to know that they are technically competent and that their passion for what they do is true and sincere are very difficult things to find. I think with at least three or four of our nurses, plus others who are developing, there is a true sense of commitment on our unit to dedicated professional oncology nursing services.

I think a lot of people here have been in other organizations, and they see the chasm that exists between our hospital and how we do business and other hospitals. It's not about the beauty of the buildings or the good food here; it really is about the people, and the 10 years I've been here, I would say that a couple of things have happened that really changed the culture, which certainly was created from the top. The way we went about this is by focusing more on people. Even how we do performance evaluations here was redone to address less performance and more service excellence, and that builds into our performance evaluation. That is a huge thing in terms of our annual reviews. We take those annual reviews very, very seriously and give very strong feedback and incentives. I've also seen that the employees that don't get it do not stay here. I think this comes from the top. It's kind of like there are people that get it. There are some people you can train, and there are other people who are just never going to get it. The people who never get it have slowly been weeded out of here because they are uncomfortable, which is huge. We don't have a big turnover here. The people who come here stay here because they are invested, and they are invested because they care. I think they care because there's a lot of pride, but they really care about the people they work with, about each other, and about our patients.

Since the closure of a hospital four miles down the road, our emergency room has been extremely busy, to the point where weekends it looks like a New York City emergency room. The nurse manager in the emergency room has been under tremendous pressure to cope with the volume, staffing, and throughput problems that exist because of that. It's been a very, very tough time in the last year, and at the same time, we've tried to get our patient satisfaction scores in the emergency room stabilized. I personally have been very supportive of her. When the scores have dipped because of tremendously high volume, I've tried to be a cheerleader and never get down on her or the staff. When the scores went up significantly, we went down and had a cake for the staff. I think that it was very important for me to show support to that department, to the staff, to the doctors, and to the nurse management team during a very, very difficult period of time. I have allocated resources and given the management team the space they need to improve operations and deal with the volume. I think knowing that the CEO of the organization is behind them 100% gives them direction and gives them confidence. I'm even having the physician director and the nurse manager come and talk to my board of directors in February about all that we've done in the emergency room to try and improve it. So I think that my support has caused them to rise to the top and really show their stuff.

I was nominated as the Helen Meehan Award recipient. It is a nursing award given on an annual basis. They select one nurse out of the entire nursing staff here who exemplifies nursing. I just felt very honored to receive that award. The administrator who gave me the award also allowed me to participate in a research course with her and another nurse manager. The course took place in Italy and was sponsored through a local university. The students from the university recognized me as a good nurse manager. The students felt they had great experiences working with me, so, the university wanted to give something back to the hospital.

I was a 24-year-old kid coming into this place. My boss took me under her belt and introduced me to the institution. Now, over the next 25 years, we built a relationship as we grew and worked together. She was always there for me, but on the flip side, I was always there for her. In this relationship we built, we virtually knew what the other needed done before it was even done. So it was almost one hand washing the other. Over the years and even today the relationship that we have is a special one.

It's hard to work in isolation here. This is a team spirit sort of place. If you realize all of the resources available to you here, there is always something somebody can do for you. There is a feeling that anything that needs to be done can be done in this hospital. We are like a town. We have food service. We have chaplains, doctors, and carpenters, and we've got everything a town could possibly want. It's a learning town. We are constantly enriching ourselves. We constantly have classes going whether it's management training or nursing grand rounds. Everybody is always learning, and the hospital supports that. It's part of the service excellence atmosphere. We are trying to better ourselves so that we can be the best we can be for our patients. I love that. I wish I could take more. There is so much here to take advantage of. Why would you want to work anywhere else?

I am very challenged in terms of the work that's expected of me. It really makes me reach. I'm always looking to improve my skills. I'm involved in different kinds of projects and exploring challenging opportunities. I happen to gain a lot of professional satisfaction from that.

First-Class Service

From the moment that you arrive at Greenwich Hospital you believe that you are either in the Ritz or The Four Seasons, and you get confused. Why? Because there is music that immediately hits you when you walk in the door. The music comes from a piano. You enter an atrium that seems like three stories high. You notice immediately that you don't have the feeling, the aroma, or the sound of a hospital. To me that's appealing; it calms people down.

Then someone at the front desk approaches you. Everyone, from the volunteers at the front of the hospital to the physicians and nurses, has smiles on their faces and a very, very positive attitude. Now I've been very fortunate myself for when my kids have had to come here. It was nothing real serious, but I can imagine if you go in there with a serious problem how comforting it is.

Greenwich is like no other hospital. The people who work there, the nurses and the nonprofessionals, are like no other. Even the person that comes into your room to sweep asks permission to come into the room, and they keep the place immaculate. You don't think you are in a hospital. The food is absolutely incredible, like no other hospital. I'm going to tell you my own experience. My doctor discharged me at 11:00 a.m., and he said I could go home. I said, "I'm not going to go home yet. I'm going to stay for lunch." He asked me what I was having for lunch. I waited for the tray to come up, and there it was. I felt like I was in a first-class restaurant. The food is to die for, not literally though.

I have been in a number of hospitals in New York City and New England because of my wife's treatments and operations. The parking at Greenwich Hospital is excellent. There is valet parking. The attendants are very courteous. They help put patients in wheelchairs. The waiting area is also exceptional; a five-star hotel lobby is not as comfortable and pleasant. The color lithographs in the waiting area, in the corridors, and in the patients' rooms are the most cheerful pictures you can imagine. Most of these depict the sunny Riviera. Just looking at them, one is immediately in a better mood. They even ask the patients whether they like the picture in their room. If not, they offer another.

This organization is excellent and efficient and better than anywhere else I know. The checking-in area is on the balcony overlooking the grand piano. There are two restaurants—one is cafeteria style, and one is a cafe. The food is very good, and the most courteous personnel serve it. Finally, I should mention the patients' rooms; they are all single-bed rooms and are almost like a five-star hotel room. One doesn't feel like you are in a hospital!

My employees do much more than smile and provide information. They are very aware that first impressions are everything in this business, and they are very aware of their actions and surroundings.

One neonatologist is phenomenal. With his own money, he takes a picture of every single NICU baby for the parent. He prints the picture with their name on it. He does it quietly. No one says anything about it. If the mom is still in bed and can't be wheeled in to the NICU to see her baby, he brings this picture to her. Then before they go home, he takes another picture, puts it in an envelope for them and writes, "Good luck." There is also a volunteer that knits a blanket for every single one of those NICU babies.

We had an older patient here who lived across the street in the apartment building. She had a housekeeper. Well unfortunately, the patient's house-keeper ended up in the bed next to her. When they were both getting dis-charged, the chief clinical dietitian came to me and said, "Listen, these two are going home, and they have no way to take care of themselves. Can we do something? Can I get them meals?"

I said, "All right, let's think about it." So we put together a plan. We got the transporters through downstairs. I got the chef together, and we produced meals—lunch and dinner for these two ladies. We hand delivered them to their apartment for 10 to 15 days while they were both recuperating until they got back on their feet. We did that at no charge to the patients. We pro-vided the service, and in the end, the people responsible for the two ladies sent roses to everybody who was involved.

Employee Initiative and Engagement

From the COO perspective, I'll give you an illustration of employee initiative. It had to do with needle sticks: how many times it took a nurse or a technician to stick the patient in order to draw blood or to start an IV. We saw a number of complaints, so we created a team who went off and did their thing. They retrained the staff. They changed the policy and procedure and changed the bore of the needle. Sure enough, the number of complaints started to go down. We went on for about a year and a half with very few complaints.

Then one day there seemed to be three or four complaints. At the end of the weekly steering committee meeting, I said, "Has anything changed in all of this?" Nobody said anything. So I got back to my office, and here was an e-mail from one of the nurse managers. She said, "The needles have been back-ordered by the manufacturer. Do you think there is any relationship to what's going on?"

I sent that down to materials management and asked them to check into it. Several days later I was walking through the hospital making rounds. I walked through one of the employee lounge areas, and an employee walked up to me and said, "I think I've solved your problem. The needles have been back-ordered. I called the company and the next time they get an order they will send us the first shipment they have. I also called another hospital, and they had an extra supply. They shipped them over to fill in the gap until we get those from the manufacturer."

I extended my appreciation to him. I said, "Thanks. That was great thinking. I really appreciate what you did." Inside I was just having a riot! I was so excited because what was happening here is that this guy on the loading dock is looking at his job in terms of what the nurse was doing upstairs. It was an illustration of bringing our organization together in providing excellent care to the patients that come to Greenwich Hospital.

We delivered a rose on every dinner tray the evening after a fire alarm went off for 20 minutes in the middle of the night.

We were building a new building right next to the existing one. There were nine rooms up against the new construction area. Some of the rooms were pediatric rooms. It meant that 18 beds would look right onto the new building under construction. You can imagine what a pleasant site it was seeing the guys bending over. So, we put a wall up to separate the new rooms from the old.

The wall took on a life of its own. We got painters to paint it sky blue. Then someone said, "Wouldn't it be neat if we had the lights go off at 7 p.m. and go on again at 7 a.m. to simulate the sun coming up and going down?" So we had a timer installed. Someone noticed that when you look down from the rooms you see the crummy concrete. One of the guys went to Home Depot and bought some Astroturf and rolled the Astroturf out there so it looked kind of like a garden. Someone else said, "You know what would really look nice on that blue wall is some clouds." One of the painters is also an artist. He went out there and painted the nicest clouds you can imagine. They weren't just white; they had definition. It really turned out to be a great experience.

We sealed off the space and put up cards saying, "Please enjoy the simulated sunlight." The patients liked the simulated outdoors. We got the children plastic hard hats, which they enjoyed. The benefit to us was that we got to use the rooms close to the construction site for a lot longer than we had imagined. The funny part was that the State Department of Health and Joint Commission inspected us during that period of time. The inspectors walked into those rooms overlooking the construction site and didn't even say a word. We didn't receive any negative comments. It wound up being a team success. We really took a negative experience and turned it around.

We have a lot of fun in the service excellence committee. We keep the Top 10 List, based on Art Linkletter's "Kids Say the Darndest Things." We keep track of funny things patients say on their patient feedback forms like, "Would you please paint double-solid lines in the connecting corridor between the buildings to remind people to stay on their own side! I just got run over by a doctor!" and "The celebration dinner was nice, but the champagne just had too many bubbles. Could you get better champagne?" The purpose is not to make fun of patients but to use this as a way to include humor in the committee meetings. There is a lot of wisdom in a lot of things the patients say.

In our department, when we have a big thing, we get everybody involved. We had a young man here in oncology with leukemia. His young wife had just delivered their first baby. The patient was able to go to labor and delivery and be there at the birth. Two days later mom and baby are ready to go home, but dad is not ready to go home. The patient's nurse was sitting down at lunch and briefly explained this patient's situation. "I was thinking about something. What if they had a web cam? Can we rig it up somehow?"

"Um, I don't know, but I know who to call." I called our IS department. I went to one particular guy who's fabulous, and I said, "Teach me about web cams. What do you need to do? Do you know how? Can you watch on the Internet?"

"For what? What are you thinking here?"

So I started to explain the story. If you want to get buy in from everybody, you need to explain the story as if it was your story or theirs. So I explained the story and he said, "Oh, I see. So if we set up a web cam at home, he could see his baby all of the time. You know what? I've got a brand new web cam here that we were going to use for something else, but I can delay that if you want. You have to configure a computer to the right settings. It would probably be easier if we took this extra laptop that I have here. I could set it up here and then take it over to their home."

Then we called the folks from the TV system and said, "Can we do this?" Once we figured out that we could do it, we went to the wife and said, "This is what we're thinking."

She said, "You've got to be kidding."

IS went over to the wife's apartment here in Greenwich within 24 hours of a nurse asking "what if?" They set up the web cam, showed the wife how to work it, and within 24 hours dad saw his new baby on television. We gave this dad 2:00 a.m. feedings that he never got home for. We gave him a few more minutes with his child. He died a couple of weeks later here in the hospital.

Defining Moments

Last summer we faced a very difficult decision of deciding to close our home care division and transitioning our patients to another home care agency. We were losing a million to a million and a half dollars a year. We just could no longer sustain it. We had to decide how we would communicate that decision. I had spent a lot of time thinking about whether or not this was the right thing to do. A former VP of nursing who worked here used to always say, "You know, if you're making the decision for the right reasons, then it's probably the right decision."

The people didn't know about this. So going into the meeting, I thought about the impact this was going to have on people's lives. We had kept it confidential. There would be surprise, anger, and frustration. People would become emotional. I thought about all of this stuff.

We talked to the staff first because we wanted to get our rationale out there. We communicated directly to the staff telling them: This is what happened. This is why we have to do this. This is the background. These are the resources that are here to help you. This is what we're going to do to transition you out, and all of our resources are here to help. The hospital did the right thing, communicated the right way. The human resources people spent hours working with the staff. We were able to transition everybody into another job. Some of them retired. Some of them moved into other positions here. Some of them went elsewhere. I believe that everyone who wanted to work found a job. So we are trying to do the right thing for the right reasons in the right way.

Somebody once told me that trust is defined as predictability. In our organization we felt that trust was so important that we had to do things differently than you would conventionally do. We provide predictability for our staff. I think our staff has respect for the organization. There's no murmuring. There's no carrying on like, "What did they do?" The hospital does the right thing, communicates the right way.

We exist for the purpose of caring for patients. I think that becomes the standard by which we try to measure the decisions that we are making, and sometimes that's really hard. You've got financial pressures, and you've got all kinds of other pressures that are happening. I think to me that that's what it's all about. We are here for the purpose of servicing or providing care to patients; that's why we exist.

I was out at the front desk with some of my staff one evening. We have a grand piano in the lobby with a "do not touch" sign on it. Every once in a while you have very enthusiastic children who bang on the piano. There are a couple of ways you could deal with that. You might say, "Please don't bang on the piano." Another way is to find out what's going on. So I grabbed a bottle of bubbles from the registration desk and went to investigate. There were two little girls and a mom who were roaming around, looking very worried, and not really paying attention to the girls. So I cautiously went up to the little girls and said, "Would you like to play?" I engaged the children, and when mom came over, I started to engage her. I said, "You look worried. What's happening?"

"Oh, we've had such a rough day." The mom said and began to tell their story. Two days ago she was in Europe with the two girls. She was a military woman, and she was being deployed back into a base in Rhode Island. They traveled to Washington and met her elderly father who had come from Michigan to drive up the coast to Rhode Island with them. They got as far as the George Washington Bridge when he started feeling bad. In Greenwich, they pulled off Rt. 95 to a gas station, and when he got out of the car, he couldn't stand. Dad is ill. The children have been in the car all day. So they called an ambulance, and she, with two small girls, followed the ambulance here.

They don't know Greenwich. They are tired. By the time I approached her girls they had not eaten anything except cookies all day. It is a good thing the girls were banging on the piano and kind of getting our attention. Mom was worried about her father who was being admitted to ICU, and she has a tremendous headache. She's lost in our lobby, and she doesn't know where to stay or what to do. She needed to get to the ED to see about her dad.

I told her we would help her. "If you trust me with your children, I will take them downstairs and get a good dinner for them. Here's my pager number. Have anybody page me." Then I gave her directions so that she was able to go to her father. I went downstairs and walked into the cafeteria with two little girls. People knew something was going on. "You must be involved in doing something. How can we help?" We started making things happen. The guys behind the counter in the cafeteria began working on getting something for the kids to eat. Then somebody from a completely different department said, "Can we get highchairs for you?" There was a staff recognition party going on in the back, so we gave the kids some frozen yogurt. Somebody made balloons for the kids. They think it's a big picnic. The guys in the back are packing up sandwiches for mom.

I made some phone calls and found out the dad's going to be admitted. I called up to ambulatory surgery and said, "I need some aspirin for this mom." They said, "Okay, its off protocol, but we'll sneak you some." I called our contact at the Hyatt and said, "I need a room now for as cheap as you can give it to me because I have a mom that needs it."

I went back to the mom and said, "Look, I've arranged for accommodations for you tonight. It's the Hyatt up the street. Here are some sandwiches. Here is some aspirin. How's dad? Meet me out front and I'll show you the way to the hotel." We paid for the room, $99. So what? The children were safe.

She got rest, and dad was well taken care of. The next day they ended up going on. We never heard from them again, but you can't help but wonder what impact you made on that day. I think what we do best here is respond to that type of need. That night I helped tuck two little girls into bed.

Believing in People

I am a manager of a fairly small department, and I had 10 applicants for a very important position. What I generally do first is interview the candidates myself. I ask them to tell me about their customer service background. I ask about times when they excelled in customer service and ask them to explain what they did. So we go through a fairly long, detailed interview. Then I bring them back for a second interview—a staff interview. I share with my staff what the first interview revealed and that I feel confident to bring this person back for a second interview.

We go over to the coffee shop, sit down kind of in the back corner—so it is a nonthreatening environment, and we just start chatting. I watch the candidate interacting with my staff. That's important for me to see because I want to see how that blends. Are they interacting well? Once I see that I get up and excuse myself. I let them chat.

I bring the staff back, and I ask, "What did you see? What did you like? Did you have any questions? How did the candidate react to you?" It becomes a team process of selection. I think it's such a wonderful event to create a solid team. I can think of no better way to give a new person a start in a department. The new person who is coming is going to have a wonderful start in the department because everybody was involved in the process. It wasn't just a unilateral decision.

I've had my shots at recognition. I feel terrific. I feel honored. The key is that I didn't achieve it alone. I believe that people are successful because people around them want them to be successful. I've always believed that, and I always will. That's why interpersonal skills are so important. No person can achieve anything as special as this without having a full team of people working with him or her.

An RN preceptor welcomes all new staff. At the end of their orientation, each person is presented with a welcome basket that has maps and t-shirts, gum, candy, movie tickets, etc. She also holds an annual orientation graduation for everyone who oriented that previous year.

One of my night nurses suggested we place a recognition board on the unit. Within a short period of time, that board was filled with hearts and notes of thanks and recognition to other staff members. What was fun and rewarding to me was to read the thank-yous sent to others and know that something as simple as a little note brings so much joy to my staff.

One of our coordinators, who is not a medical professional, came to see me almost two years ago. She sat down and said, "I have something to tell you. I hate the sight of blood. I pass out in patients' rooms if they start describing awful things." She really struggles with that challenge. One day we were sitting at lunch, and she said, "Oh, I have to tell you what happened in the hallway today." She went on to tell the story that somebody was coming into the emergency room entrance dripping blood from their elbow. They had their hand in a plastic bag, and it was really kind of ugly. "I brought them to the emergency room, and then I got somebody to clean up." We were all just staring at her. We can't believe she's even repeating this story much less having not passed out. Later that day, I went to the gift shop and bought this little bear with hospital scrubs on, and I paged all of the full-time staff. I said, "You guys, we've got to recognize this. This is really a kind of breakthrough for this staff member." We all went to the emergency room entrance. We hid and then paged her to that area. Once she got there, we all popped out and made it a big ceremony. We told her, "This is the stand-up award for service—great service to a patient. This was a great breakthrough for you." The bear sits on her shelf.

I took the leadership team of about 120 people off-site last Thursday and Friday. We had a wonderful day and a half talking about service excellence— going from good to wow. Everybody was energized and ready to take us to another notch. I think sometimes you get wrapped up in a lot of things. This got everybody refocused. I could tell how committed people really are.

I had a staff meeting. I brought bagels, and we gathered around the table in the staff lounge. I presented the service scores to the staff. All they could do was just sit there, clap, and say, "Oh, yes, we got that." They were very excited. I challenged them and said, "Do you think we can go to the 100th percentile next time?" The staff received it very positively.

Some people who are not directly involved in patient care did not get data on our departments. One individual asked to be informed how the hospital is doing. I said, "Wow, you're right. Thank you." You make an assumption that everybody knows what's going on, and there are some people who don't have access to the patient satisfaction reports. I was grateful to that individual for pointing that out, and I thanked him after the meeting. Then we devised a way for everybody to see data.

I came across a poem many years ago entitled *Beatitudes of a Leader*. I had it professionally printed. At the bottom I wrote, "With sincere appreciation" and my name. I've had it mounted in a frame. *Beatitudes of a Leader* sets an aspiration in terms of leadership style. On occasions I've given that certificate to key managers. It makes the statement, "Blessed are they who are flexible for they shall not be broken." It's the idea of flexibility. Having your head in the clouds and your feet on the ground. It makes people say, "Wow." My hope is that it draws them into the future, lifting their aspirations and what they want to achieve in their careers.

When we were getting ready to open this building, the group was really pulling hard. We were all working together before any of the festivities began with the open house. I invited the group out for dinner on a night when the CEO was available. We went to one of the local restaurants. These hard-working people haven't been to many of these things. I was able to publicly express my appreciation to each of them for the work that they were doing, pulling this project together, sticking to it, and paying attention to the details.

We started moving into a new building that we had been planning for 10 years. As the CEO, I saw these drawings. I had people talk to me about finishes, and I saw it being built. Then all of a sudden it was becoming a reality. As I was driving to work I was thinking there was no doubt in my mind that this move was going to go smooth as silk. No doubt in my mind. Actually, although it was a six-minute drive, I was extremely relaxed. I felt confident I felt a sense of joy, a sense of pride, and I knew that this team was made up of a wonderful group of individuals who are caring, kind, want to be successful, and want to make the organization successful. There was never any worry or concern. It was just, from my perspective, enjoyment in a way: fulfillment and pride.

When you've helped to develop something so special, you owe it to people to try and continue the special nature of the organization. The people are among the most special people that I ever worked with throughout my career.

Editor Commentary

The vision, passion, and obsession around service at Greenwich Hospital are apparent in the everyday actions of leaders, physicians, and staff throughout the organization; however, this isn't a story solely about providing customer service—it's a story about creating the link between service and the overall success of the organization—whether achieving clinical or financial results or creating the stories that drive patient and employee satisfaction. The consistent messages and actions that link their service success to overall organizational goals are impressive.

The meaningful connection of the service standards (expectations) to employee evaluations and compensation at 60% is quite a statement. Employees readily see how their everyday actions are linked to their personal success as well. The linkage of the performance goals (in service and everywhere else) to the money put into the retirement fund is brilliant.

The senior leadership has developed and implemented several structures and tools that are designed to keep service at the forefront of every staff member's mind. It starts with the Wednesday meeting—led by the CEO and COO—which reviews all of the input from patients, families, visitors, and community members received during the past week. The expectation of remedial action and accountability for results by the next week's meeting are extraordinary.

Celebrations of all sorts—formal and informal—provide inspiration and appreciation to the staff. These contribute to the development of teamwork and trust that is essential to their ongoing success. By recognizing what is going well and sharing heart-warming stories from patients and others, staff members are encouraged to continue to improve.

Leadership development has played a key role in their ongoing improvement efforts. Better leaders are better able to lead—to have the courage to empower their teams, to make results happen quickly, to remove barriers. The investment the organization makes in education for staff at all levels has created a learning organization. Staff members are constantly asking, "How can we make this better?" They recognize the need for additional knowledge and skills development and tie this to improved performance. They have asked and answered the question, "Do they think the less educated staff we have the better we are going to be able to perform?" They recognize the need for additional knowledge and skills development and tie this to improved performance.

They are, in the words of their leaders, employees, physicians, and patients, a "special place" filled with special people, empowered to make a difference every day.

Table 11-1 Organizational Demographics

Organization	Sharp HealthCare
Location	San Diego, CA
Setting	Urban
Communities served	All
Type of organization	Not-for-profit health care system
Number of beds	1,727
Number of FTEs	14,000
Organizational awards	California Awards for Performance Excellence (California Malcolm Baldrige Affiliate). 2005 Eureka Award—Silver award winner
	Named best integrated health network in California (number 1 in California and number 22 in the nation) by *Modern Healthcare* in 2006
	Named one of the Most Wired organizations for the 8th consecutive year
Focus area	Outpatient Endoscopy Unit of the Sharp Memorial Outpatient Pavilion
Focus area Best practices and awards	Consistently above the 90th percentile in patient satisfaction (Press Ganey national database) for the past 4 years
	Service on a Silver Tray
	Staff turnover for the endoscopy department is between 0% and 2%
	Employee satisfaction overall for the department is 4.73 on a 5-point scale

CHAPTER 11

Connecting to a Vision

Contributor: Lolma Olson

The stories in this chapter are the voices of the corporate CEO and members of the senior executive team at Sharp HealthCare, the CEO and at Sharp Memorial Hospital, the director and staff from the Outpatient Pavilion, a nurse manager and the staff from the endoscopy center, and their patients. Here are their stories.

SHARP HEALTHCARE

Communicating the Vision

We needed to rally our vision of being the best place to work, practice medicine, and receive care. This is my "guiding light" and is a "beacon" for myself and my co-workers.

I look very closely at the vision because it certainly elevates us organizationally in terms of its power. I see it as two things. One is it's a hope: It's an aspiration for people to share. Also, it is a point of pride. Every single employee can rally around it. They can speak to it, and they can see their part in making Sharp an awesome place.

At our all-staff assemblies, we communicate a vision to thousands of people. Although these people work different shifts all around the clock, we get everybody together. To actually bring 14,000 people together and see their energy and passion has been an absolute high. We watch them engage and then realize we can be better, as we all go on a journey to create a better organization.

When planning the The Sharp Experience all-staff assembly, we think about several key things. One is the ultimate outcome. How are we going to create this employee event in a way that continues to engage our work force? Another is how are we going to execute so that we have 14,000 people walking around saying, "Healthcare is the best industry in the world," and "Working at Sharp is the right place for me to be?" We are always thinking about how we can make sure that after an hour everybody feels like they are a participant and an owner. How can we make this great? We want people to feel like their work from the week before mattered—that it didn't get discounted or overlooked.

We needed to get our message down to the front-line staff. We had this idea for this year's all-staff assembly, and it just started rolling. Who could we ask to speak, and what would that look like? We decided to ask people from the Sharp HealthCare documentary to do the teaching and presenting. The staff would know these people from having just seen them on the screen. (We produce a video documentary to show at our assemblies.)

For example, one man who works in engineering—he calls himself Motorhead Mike—creates special adaptations for patients out of pieces and parts. At one point someone said, "We want this woman who is a burn victim to be able to apply make-up. She cannot do it the regular way." So Motorhead Mike created a foot-pedal pump for her to apply make-up by airbrush. He was able to show the pride of someone being able to go above and beyond his regular job to help a patient. He also talked about little things like going in a patient's room and using some of The Sharp Experience five fundamentals of service. People just related to him. People just got it. It was so great. We've been able to enroll people who may not have an opportunity to really see their part in The Sharp Experience.

At our last all-staff assembly, I introduced a mother and her baby. Previously, a car had rammed this woman, who was eight months pregnant, while she was sitting at a bus stop. The baby came out unexpectedly, and they had to do CPR on the baby and the mother. In our documentary, we showed her incredible hospitalization with real footage from ER and the ICU in our attempt to save her. They both survived, and both are well. It struck me that this was an incredible result, and we could all be proud of it. It was an opportunity to point out that, if you were working in materials management, you were just as much a part of the team as the nurses, doctors, and therapists.

I told people that if there was ever a time where they were concerned about what they were doing in life, they should look at this mother and baby and know what they were a part of. You may think that you are just ordering latex gloves. Well you are, but it's much more than that. You are a part of this success just as much a part of it as those who stuck a needle in her or intubated her.

We take patient satisfaction very seriously. Staff gets involved in reviewing feedback that we get from the patients. We do follow-up phone calls with our patients to find out how their stay was. We don't rely solely on the satisfaction scores coming back. We live that vision every day.

I teach people around the system how to use the patient satisfaction data. I conduct focus groups so that we can really get people dialoguing not only about the current state of things but also about the ideal state. I use the patient's written words, positive or negative, to get people thinking from the patient's point of view. I have been known to bring patients who have been harmed in our organization to speak to our leadership teams. We've had 1,100 people sobbing after realizing what has happened because of our mistakes.

One of my most uncomfortable leadership sessions involved our leaders reading patient comments. There were 50 different voices getting up and reading patient comments. When you have the right mix of positive and not so positive comments, it is just overwhelming for people to hear.

Leadership Sets the Tone

Our manager always sets the tone for us. We all know how difficult it is to make sure that our department runs smoothly. She makes it look easy. She is fair and sets a good example for everyone.

I'm in the departments every day, generally more than once a day. So they see me. They feel comfortable with me. When there's a complaint of any kind I will follow-up on it. I think the important piece from them to hear is "we'll get back to you; we'll fix it." Then they see that it's fixed, or if it can't be fixed, I explain honestly why it can't.

One weekend about three years ago the Suzuki Marathon was in town. One of our nurses was working and resuscitated a runner from Los Angeles. The ambulance team ended up bringing him to Sharp Memorial Hospital. It turned out he was a physician from LA. He was critically ill. He needed all of the sexy things that Sharp Memorial could do to help him survive and get him better.

His family was contacted and informed of how sick he was. They were shocked. They drove down to Sharp from Los Angeles. Their directions took them by the freeway, and they saw the big Sharp sign outside the door. They got off the freeway and were trying to get in the building to see their husband and father, but all the doors were locked. They didn't realize this was an administration building. While they were pounding on the doors and ringing the doorbell, a gentleman drove up in a truck and asked what they were doing. After hearing the story, the gentleman explained to them that they were in the wrong place. They really needed to be at Sharp Memorial Hospital, which is only a mile or two away. While he's trying to explain to them where to go, it becomes clear to him the state of mind that this family is in. "This ain't going to work." So he got in his truck and drove them over.

One of our nurses heard this story and decided she was going to track down the person who brought them over. She tried to figure out if it was one of the environmental services people or more likely one of the IT people that comes in to check on things every now and then. It turned out that it was our CEO. He came in because he had left some papers in the office. It was really impressive to see that our boss, who really is an incredible guy, do something like that, not because it's the Sharp way but because it was the right thing to do.

Set the tone

The Right Fit

It was the way the staff behaved, the quality of people they have. They made me feel important.

I take care to get the right people that fit into this unit. In other words, I select people who really show compassion and caring and a real love of patients. I think that's truly a great part of our success—that we have the right people in this department. What's important for me is that they have a positive attitude and that they are really highly motivated people. Anybody can learn the technical stuff, but you can't teach the attitude. You can't teach compassion. You can't teach a high level of motivation.

I had the opportunity to hire the right people and be very clear about what our expectations were for great service. We handpicked 90 staff that joined us from other parts of our organization. We hired the best of the best.

When we hire people, we're really looking for customer service skills. One of the things we learned on this journey is that if you don't come to us with customer service ingrained within you we can't teach you. We have worked with some individuals for a long time; we really wanted them to get it. We found generally if they don't display it in an interview we can't get there. It's really not a great "aha" when you think about it. The tuck and the tack in the RN and the professional areas and the people who are actually doing the clinical work are one thing, but when you've got front-line staff who are greeting and interacting with patients, what happens if they don't have those skills?

We don't tolerate poor customer service, and we have let staff go for that reason. So it's very clear in the staff's mind that this is our environment. I think because of that we have a group of staff who like each other and like working here. They want to work in that kind of environment. That's who they are. That's the person they are. I feel very fortunate because of that, and that's what's playing into the success that we're having—it's got to be.

When I interview someone, I have two other colleagues in the interview with me, and together we share our impressions. We ask them to give examples of what they've done in the past. Then we ask ourselves, "Will this person fit in? Does this person have the right attitude? Does this person have the commitment to the unit, to the organization? Do they seem real enough to want to be here? Do we have a good feeling about them?" This last impression is hard to articulate, but you know it when you see it. If we can't say yes to all of these questions, we don't hire them. We don't hire for potential because we know that "what you see is what you get."

People knew that I would be the perfect candidate for this position because I care about patients; I know how to interact with patients. You know. A lot of times I put myself in their position. How would I want to be treated if I were in their shoes? I would treat them with respect and caring. I thank God for my colleagues because without them I wouldn't have a big family.

There are some people you can't teach to be "this way." It's almost like these people have been screened to already be good with people. I think that if someone didn't fit in here, they wouldn't be here very long. It would be recognized because it would put a snag into their program. People know how to treat people here. They have great teamwork, and they obviously work on it. They give complete care.

We interviewed a receptionist. I was interested in the fact that she was very interested in what we had to say, and she asked a lot of questions. When I talked about our philosophy here in endoscopy, it was something that she wanted to be a part of and was excited during the interview. Those are the pieces that I look for: They want to contribute something to the department. She asked questions about how her role would fit into this philosophy, and she told me what she was willing to do and what she would like to do. She was really eager. I asked her, "When do you want to start?" I look for that hunger. I just want somebody really truly compassionate about what they do. I am just grateful that she is here. I thank her every day for taking care of the group and me.

Two years into the building we had lost an endoscopy tech who was very close to the physicians. I got a lot of pressure from physicians about the person who was leaving. He had been in my department for a number of years, and we relied quite heavily on him. Although he was close to the physicians, he sort of diminished nursing by cutting nurses down in front of physicians. To me, it was not healthy for the group. While he had a lot of talent and was very close to physicians, it didn't make sense for me to keep somebody here who ruined the morale of the staff. It wasn't in line with what we wanted to do at the pavilion. He was a lovely person. He just was not supportive of what I felt was important here. That ultimately led to his leaving. The physicians sort of pushed the issue and said, "He needs to come back." They didn't understand, and they were certain we would not be successful without him. Because of our commitment we just sort of turned it all around.

Despite this issue, our physicians are interested in becoming partners with the organization and are interested in bringing in more business to this department. They are sending patients from other hospitals here; they decided to close some of their business down at the other places to come here, and to me—that was a success of the whole group.

My manager wrote a letter to our director, and that helped me out a lot. I ended up becoming full time because they recognized that I was doing my job. They recognized that I was going out of my way, and I didn't do it because I wanted to become full time. I did it because that's just me. I talk to the people. When there are patients sitting in the lobby, I go and sit down and talk to them because I understand they're bored. I make sure they feel at home, and my manager loves the idea of that. I communicate with the patients. Whether it's the patients or the family members, I let them know, " I want you to feel like you're at home. If you fall asleep, it's okay; you're here for hours."

Five-Star Journey

The outpatient pavilion opened three years ago. Prior to that point, I had the opportunity of bringing together staff who would work in this building. I really think that this was one of the highest points in my career; with this opportunity of creating an environment and having such huge success, it is so clear and so evident. When you look at the principles of leadership and management, they're obvious.

When I was hired, the idea of having a new building was more than just walking into some facility. We wanted people who walked in here to be impressed with more than just the building itself, but feel, "Wow, this was a great experience." I feel so strongly about customer service and outcomes, and I was really excited about being able to implement that vision. I couldn't say this is exactly how we're going to do it, but I knew it had to come from the people that were working here. At the very same time, I was hired the week that they kicked off The Sharp Experience, so Sharp itself was beginning this journey.

We created the five-star service vision, and it was very much a collaborative, participative approach. The vision itself with actual employees being a part of it was maybe the two to three months prior to opening. We started down the road and meshed some of the approaches that the The Sharp Experience had with what we were already doing.

We looked at our first entry point with the patient through to the point of care and follow-up. Where were those places along the line that we could have problems, and what would we do if those problems occurred? So we mapped the process with the staff, and then we zeroed in on intervention. We began talking about the five-star experience and how do we really want to come across. Every person came up with suggestions, both one on one and in groups. We had a number of ideas about operations and how it would be efficient in workflow. Some things worked, and some didn't.

Truly we had the opportunity to create a new culture. We knew we had a philosophy, here at the outpatient pavilion, of the five-star experience and world-class care. I made time to talk with every staff member and had staff meetings about what was important to them and what they wanted to see in the department. They brought forth their ideas. I wanted to make sure that these ideas were implemented prior to opening. There are a number of things we did to define that vision, but it was the staff themselves who created it and implemented it.

Early on, our marketing spiel for the outpatient pavilion opening was "real-class care, five-star service," and we articulated that from the day we opened. I did the orientation for staff when we first hired them. We talked about what makes five-star and had the staff articulate when they went to a hotel or when they went to a restaurant, what was different about that facility. We talked about, "Have you been to a Ritz Carlton versus Holiday Inn?" They did that. This five-star experience then took off. We talked about the fact that it's not just the way we greet people and The Sharp Experience 5 must haves—you know, that you smile and you introduce yourself, take people where they need to go—but it's also how we interact with each other.

One of the things we did with one of our first-line staff—like the concierge, the reception staff, and anyone who is greeting people—is to have them visualize what a five-star experience is. I actually took them all on field trips to hotels in the community, and they had to rank the hotels on a whole variety of areas. They were asked to describe the differences: What was it about that five-star hotel that separated it from anything else? What is it about our department that we can do that makes it a five-star experience?

I had a whole long list of things to look for when we went to hotels. What did they look like? How did they greet us? We'd sit in lobbies watching and writing on notepads. At that point, we already had defined some of the scripting and some of the behaviors we expected, so then when they were looking at others, they had something to judge them by. We came back together, and I facilitated a retreat. I videotaped them in role playing so that they could critique themselves on their appearances, whether they smiled, and how they greeted people. We did role playing to define what we thought greetings should look like.

I would pretend I was admitting a patient, and we would go through scripting and saying good morning, smiling, and shaking hands. I would give the staff guidelines on how to behave with patients. This wasn't hard for them because I took care to get the right people that fit into this unit. They really show compassion and caring and a real love of patients, and I think that's a great part of our success.

We looked for service recovery. We videotaped staff and saw that they weren't smiling when they thought they were. We also talked about hotel rooms. If you went into a hotel room and there was hair in the bathroom and if there were things in wastebasket, what would you do? From the beginning, we dressed all of the front staff in their navy blazers. We talked about the fact that it's not the blazer that's making you an exceptional employee, but it makes a statement to the public. It kind of gives you that hotel concierge feel. It helps the public identify you as registration clerks and concierges.

My role was to guide them through that process to make sure we stuck to what we were committed to. I had to make sure that they had the tools and whatever they needed to be able to meet those behavior standards. For example, if I said to them that we were going to be offering patient's juice in stemmed glassware on a silver tray, I better make sure I have that silver tray and stemmed glassware on day 1, not on day 14. If I wanted to make sure that people were not eating and drinking at the nurse's station, I better make sure that doesn't happen every day. So I was either guiding them into this new behavior or supporting them through this behavior.

In other words, there was a competency that we developed about what our behavior was supposed to be like. We developed these competencies and behaviors through collaboration with the staff. What types of behaviors were important in a five-star experience? What was the unit going to look like? How were we going to conduct ourselves in front of patients and toward each other? We wanted people who were friendly and positive and willing to serve. I felt that if we came to this department and tried to implement a behavior change after the opening it would be more difficult. In other words, it was important for me that we had this attitude change before we opened so that we were already doing it when we opened. This ties into our Sharp Experience and our behavior standards, so it was really nothing new. It was implementing it in a five-star way, if you will.

If somebody is not happy, my concierge is always giving free parking. I think that every staff person is very comfortable with doing this. It's clearly a Sharp HealthCare kind of thing. Doing a lot of service recovery is not seen as a negative thing. They have to account for what they've given away, but it's not considered a negative. It's not like, "Oh my gosh. We're using too many of these things." We go through patient representatives, and risk management will write off bills and attribute them to a satisfied customer.

I think the peak experience is that they are actually living it. They are doing it not because of me; it was because they wanted to. It's just so routine now. The staff really determined what kind of caregivers they wanted to be and what kind of service they wanted to provide. They want to work in that kind of environment. That's who they are. That's the person they are. I feel very fortunate because of that, and that's what's playing into the success that we're having. It's got to be. You could stop and talk to any staff here. They know what is expected of them, how they interact, how we treat people.

Every day I see my staff enjoying their patients and having a good time. I think it's very satisfying for the nursing staff. So that to me has a lot to do with satisfaction. They're able to work with patients with ease, and patients leave and say, "Gosh this wasn't so bad at all. I love you all." The patients write notes; they send us candy and, that kind of gratitude sort of feeds itself.

As for sustaining this great service, I have no question in my mind that it will be sustained. I think if someone attempted to stop it, there would be a big rebellion. It would be difficult to stop the ball from rolling because it's a part of the staff's being, their belief system, and their value structure. They own it. It's not just management dictating you must do it this way. They are going to continue it on, and they would be hard pressed if you brought a manager in who tried to stop them from doing it.

It's pretty amazing really because the patients only come in for an hour. They get so much special treatment that they don't want to leave. One thing we do after the procedure is give them what we like to call appetizers or a big lunch because it's going to be their first meal of the day, and it tickles them. I can tell. We give them a silver tray, and there's a champagne glass.

First of all, what impresses me is that they treat us like people in a five-star hotel. They are a well-oiled machine.

It was the most unbelievable experience I've ever had. It was very pleasant, and the people were just magnificent.

Everything is done at the right time. It's just the way they handle you, the way they move around, and the caring conversations they have with you.

I thought the volunteer that met me at the entrance that morning was the sweetest person. She had on a pleated skirt and a blue blazer. I felt so much like I was at a five-star hotel.

Communication is a big deal. They call you by your name. That's important. Then there is the one that calls you afterward to be sure you're okay.

Nobody wants a colonoscopy, but you just forgot that's why you were there. They made it like a party. I felt so much like I was in a five-star hotel.

Coaching and Being Coached

We are dedicated to developing leaders in a way that we've never been committed to before. It is the underpinning of our success.

I stay here because of my relationship with our CEO. I have an extraordinary working relationship with him, and I value and respect his leadership. I have a sense of great compatibility between his strengths and weaknesses and my own strengths and weaknesses. They are complementary. He is a unique individual and a great leader. We had synergy from the start. We learned together. He does not micromanage me, and he has the ability to assess where he wants us to take risks. He is humble and is able to say when he is wrong and then move on, not wallow in it. His philosophy works: "Let's learn from our mistakes and not go there again."

I think it is really important for a leader to know their staff and have them see that you do respect them and value them. So, in my relationships with my staff and my managers, they feel that they can come to me with issues and problems and that we will problem solve together. If they come to me with something and want my help, I critique what's right and wrong, and I guide them.

I find that there are staff that need coaching, and I think, "How can I make sure that this won't happen again, and how can we be sure that this behavior has been taken care of?" One employee assured me in the beginning that she had changed, but I believe under stress her bad behavior came out again. She was cranky and snippy and said the wrong things. So I took her to the back and counseled her. I said, "I'm not sure if you want feedback about your performance, but this is what I'm observing. This is what others are observing. Are you aware of it?" She was not. Basically, we tried to talk about why it happened again and what factors played into it. She acknowledged that she had been working more hours, and she wanted to go to part time. She is working full time right now. So I sort of encouraged her to do a couple of things: to go to employee counseling, to cut back on her hours, and to approach people about her communication skills and get feedback. She asked for my support in asking others to be real honest about bad communications with her and to report it to her right away. So there was a game plan.

I think when she or any manager comes to me it's okay. If there is a problem, I think, "What can I do to help facilitate resolution of that problem?" I had a concern for her. My role was to assist her in problem solving, reaching to help her, and then supporting her in that.

Physicians don't get it yet in terms of consumer/patient satisfaction. Most physicians think, and I certainly did for a longtime, that the only thing you had to do was be a good doctor and give good care. If the person wasn't satisfied with that, it was their problem. What they don't get is that high-quality medicine is just the price of admission. You bring that to the table. That just lets you get into the sandbox. Then you have to learn all of these other skills if you really want to succeed today. Patient satisfaction is one of them. It's not the only one, but it's one of them. What I try and do is work on the attitude of my colleagues. I tell them that I know that you're a good doctor. You're a great doctor, but so is he, and so is he, and so is he. When you come in and you examine somebody without pulling the curtain around, that was okay maybe 20 years ago. It wasn't okay 10 years ago, but it's certainly not okay today. Somebody is going to complain about it. Don't be crazy. Pull the curtain.

Believing in People

The Sharp Experience isn't just about making an organization better, but it is about helping people be better people and being able to learn and grow as a person.

As CEO, I talk about the organization and what we have. The thing that makes us special is the people. It makes me feel good to be able to talk and stand up in front of the people and thank them for what they do and how they helped create the organization that we have.

I got a letter about a bunch of people who came in because there was a flood in the central supply sterile processing room one night. Everybody was called in because they had to reprocess all of the surgical supplies to be able to start surgery the next morning. I wrote a thank you card to everybody who had come back in and thanked each person for making a difference and going above and beyond. After one of the sterile processing guys got his letter, he said, "I'll never leave Sharp HealthCare because my CEO wrote that thank you note."

Our CEO is very good with compliments and with recognition. We had a very difficult situation about a year and half ago with a fairly difficult family. It wasn't going well. It was one of those things. No matter what anybody did with this particular patient, it went to hell in a hand basket. At the end of the day, we got through it, and the patient got through it. The family actually sent a nice note to our CEO outlining some of the goods and bads and highlighting the role that I played with the family in a positive way. Our CEO told me how much he appreciated what I did and then was magnanimous enough to point that out to other people. That really made a difference to me.

As a physician, I lead with my heart and receive things with my heart. To live and lead with my values means that I have been able to open up possibilities for people, to be able to passionately paint a vision for folks so that they understand about being a real leader. Role modeling is also important, and so it's about doing that which we ask others to do. This has been critical in our ability to hardwire and achieve results. Also, I value learning, and it's all about learning.

I learned that you can lead from in front: There's a time and a place for that. You can lead from behind: There's a time and a place for that, but a leader is always in the middle. A leader is always a part of the team, and there are times with you need to walk ahead. There's a time when you need to be behind.

We did a great thing where we brought in the American College of Physician Executives. Each doctor looked at a business balance sheet, looked at marketing in healthcare, looked at IT in healthcare, and looked at quality in healthcare. To me, that is leading from behind. People don't realize you're doing it. People don't necessarily even know its being done to them, but at the end of the day, I think you have to be proud as a cheerleader, as somebody who is only going to go in the direction that we should be going.

I send everybody involved thank you notes to their homes. I remember an employee thanking me afterward and her expressing how much it meant to her. In particular, I remember being able to be very specific in her thank you note about what she did. She said how much it meant to her. Recently, she received a five-year pin. She said she used to make fun of people who got them and wore them, but now it means a lot to her. She wears it.

Most important is how we recognize staff. An example of this is that one of our staff members had just reached her five years with Sharp. We gathered everybody around, and I rang this wind chime. We all clapped. In the beginning, I made a big deal of it, and then everybody began to realize the importance of acknowledging and congratulating. I was truly proud of their accomplishments. I wanted to make sure that they understood that it was important. I want to make sure that everybody plays a part in acknowledging somebody's strengths and special qualities or achievements. It is necessary to do that at work and to show your peers who understand what you do.

My manager is a great leader because she lets us be. If she feels like she needs to step in, she will, but she respects us enough to let us figure it out. She gets her point across. She walks quietly but she carries a big stick.

This morning I had a long drive in. I walked in, and there was a plate of chocolate chip cookies in recognition of work I had done. Later, my manager came out with my sapphire pin. You may notice that I don't wear any other pins, but I'm so proud of this one. It was the way she presented it to me and clapped and everything. It's wonderful to stay here for five years. In ten years, I'll get the one with two sapphires.

It's the "wows" that we get from things like the "catch me carings." Patients can write up how they've interacted with us and how we've helped them and what their experience was while they were here for their appointment. It's entered into a box, and then the director of the building will reward us. After you receive a certain amount of wows, you receive another extraordinary gift, a certificate, or a movie.

Work Family

This is the best job, when everything is lumped into that one basket, that I've ever had. I've been paid more in San Diego at other jobs, but this is by far the most satisfying thing that I've done. I just wouldn't trade it for anything.

I appreciate that my co-workers listen. I greatly appreciate that because sometimes I go home and I have no one who will listen to me. My daughter, I can talk to her, but there are certain things I cannot talk to her about, so I'd say that they're like a family to me now.

I consider them my family because I know if I have a problem I can come and talk to them anytime without feeling like they will go out and share with everyone.

Sharp cares for their employees. I don't know if you know that Sharp has an employee hotline that I think is great. If you have a down day you can call that number and talk to somebody. Sharp understands that we're here to do our job, but they also understand that we are people outside of our job and that sometimes we need someone to talk to. I love that.

My grandfather was in endoscopy two months ago. I just loved that when I told my co-workers that my grandfather was here they treated him just like they would treat any other patient. They were all very nice to my grandpa since my grandpa had dialysis. It was very hard for them to find his vein, so they got another nurse to come and help. He started getting teary eyed. So one of the nurses came and held his hand and told him that everything was going to be okay. They were trying to talk to him in Spanish because he's Spanish speaking. I like that. They were there for him. I got the goose bumps when my grandfather told my whole family, "I got good care, and my granddaughter is good at what she does." That made me feel good.

We are sincere. We don't do this Willy Nilly. You can get into recognition programs where you're throwing thank you cards at everybody, left, right, and center, but here it is sincere. Once, at one of our all-staff meetings, I did the pledge of allegiance. I asked if I could do it because I had become a citizen three or four days before. Most of them were lucky enough to be born here. I asked those who weren't born here who are now citizens to put their hand up with me in front of the other people. I bet I got 200 or 300 little thank-you cards or little notes at that time, all sincere. It was people saying, "Congratulations, glad to have you on that team."

Thanking Patients

We were really impressed with the service in all areas and then the thank you note at the end; we just couldn't believe it!

The staff got together and said, "Wouldn't it be neat if we sent thank you cards to our patients?" At the time, they were a small surgery center with four operating rooms. We now have ten operating rooms, and we are doing almost

1,000 cases a month. We carried the thank-you note idea over to this building, and then all of the other departments started doing it. It is a very simple, easy thing to do that has a dramatic impact on the patient and how they feel.

Right from the start we got thank-you cards and things we needed to write them. People were really "wowed" by that and still comment about that. I'll meet someone in the community, and they say, "Do you know that I really received a thank you and it was signed?" Everyone who interacts with the patient signs the card: even the doctor, the housekeeper, and the registration person. Anyone that had contact with the patient signs the card.

One hundred percent of our patients receive a thank-you note, and it's signed individually by those people that have actually touched the patient. It is now mailed to the patient at home and sent at the end of their procedure day.

There was a patient in a bakery in Pacific Beach. He had just had an endoscopy, and he's telling the person who worked there about his experience: "I didn't want to have this procedure, but I went. I couldn't believe it. It was amazing. They had this little silver tray. It was so fabulous, and the real amazing thing was three days later I got a thank you note that was signed by all of the caregivers and the physicians." There was a physician's wife in the bakery who was overhearing this whole thing. She went back to her husband and said, "Why aren't you writing thank-you notes?"

Last Monday we had a patient. Friday her husband came in, and he said as he's walking by, "'Hi everybody. I'm looking forward to getting my little message."

The thank-you note was hilarious. Each nurse had written a personal note on it, and one of the messages was "thank you for sharing your day with us." Three out of the five comments were hilarious. It wasn't meant to be funny, but it was like, don't they remember why I was there? I probably called five or six people to tell them about it, and I actually wrote about it in a couple of e-mails. I couldn't let it go.

Spirit of Caring

Sharp is all about patient care, so to me, my number one goal is to be there for the people and to let them know I care.

I know with Sharp it's not about bringing money—it's about patients. That's what attracted me to this company.

There was a woman who speaks English, but it's not her first language. I felt it was really important for me to be there and to extend my hand to her and let her know that Sharp was going to take good care of her.

If there were any gold medals given it should be given to the people that did my colon. You know what? They touch you. They have their hand on your arm. It feels good.

I'd like to tell about a time I was a patient here. My son dropped me off, and at the time, he was under doctor's care too. He was kind of sick and his leg was swollen, and he was on medication. The nurse told him, "Why don't you go lay down or something. We'll take good care of your mother." So he went back to the car, and he slept the whole time. When I was done, the nurse walked me all the way to the car. It was amazing. Later, she was so sweet when she called me to see how I was doing. She even wanted to know how my son was.

I had a procedure done. My sister brought me here so she dropped me off and went for a couple of errands and came back. Everything went so smoothly, and they were very prompt. I was impressed. The physician made jokes. He went and got me a warm blanket himself. It was very comfortable considering what I was there for.

My physician was just wonderful. He talked to me during the procedure. He was just perfect. In the office before the visit he was so thorough to tell me what would happen. He told me what would happen if the results were not good. He was very thorough in explaining everything. I felt very knowledge-able, and I felt that way throughout the procedure.

Well, during the deal, I was out there, you know for polyps. He told me I must have a farm of polyps. He started counting them. It was nine the first time, and then I came back last December and had five more. So he says, "You're growin 'em. I'll see you again next year." He was a great doctor. He let my wife stay with me until they rolled me in.

They welcomed me when I came in. They checked to see if I was warm enough and brought me a blanket. They never left my side. One of the nurses was there all of the time and got to know me. Then they called me after I went home the next day to follow up and sent me a beautiful card. The concern and the consideration were something else. It made me feel important. It was the way people were, the quality of the people they have there. They have their hand on your arm while they tell you what they are going to do. I was very impressed and felt cared for by everyone.

When the nurse took me back for the procedure, she asked me a few questions about myself, not about me medically, but about me as a person. Then she said she would be with me the entire time. I was then moved to another room, and she wasn't there. She came in soon after and apologized that she couldn't be with me because there had been an emergency, and she had to go take care of another person. Then she introduced me to the nurse who was going to take her place. I didn't feel like I was dropped off and left. I really liked that she introduced me to this other nurse. I felt that I was still in good hands and didn't feel like I had been switched around and moved around. There was no confusion about it. It was good.

In endoscopy, every day is a success because we help our patients as much as we can. We go out of our way because we chose to and because we care.

I remember one morning when I admitted an older patient for a procedure. When I went to the admitting lobby to bring him back for his procedure, his siblings—two sisters and one brother—stood up to accompany him. Usually we do not have the family accompany the patient because of the size of the recovery area, but I let them join us. We formed a parade: our patient, his sisters, his brother, and me. The other staff members gave me a funny look but did not interfere. I found chairs for the siblings, got the patient ready for his procedure, explained to the family what to expect, and went on to the next patient. The staff members were just amazed by this family, how they took care of one another, and were there for each other and still lived together in one home.

Several days later, our lead shared with me a comment sent to the hospital by the oldest sister. She said how well her family was treated and how professional I was. I made sure they were comfortable, knew what to expect, and made them feel validated. This is an example of how patients and their families may not know our role in the organization but expect us to function as if we were Sharp HealthCare. I felt I had done a good job representing my organization and received gratification and contentment for a job well done.

I always make sure that the patient is aware when they're going to be called. I make sure I communicate with them because they could be sitting in our waiting room for 10 minutes wondering, "Are they going to call me next?" So I always make sure that if they haven't been called, I go back and check how much longer they will have to wait. I make sure the patient knows what's going on so that they're not waiting and thinking that we're neglecting them or forgot about them. I communicate with family members also. I try to speak to them every half an hour and let them know how the family member is doing.

There's one patient I remember that was going to have a birthday the following day. He was older. He had been at Pearl Harbor. This was right around Pearl Harbor Day. He did not have any family nearby and was really lonely. He said at home he hardly ever gets dressed. We found out it was his birthday, and we ended up singing happy birthday and got him a piece of cake. He loved it. We didn't have any candles, so we made candles out of paper towels.

I comfort people as I'm walking them to the department because people are concerned and worried, you know. I comfort them before we actually get there, before they do any registering or anything like that. I share with them my experience when I came here for the same procedure. That experience really brings to light how wonderful that department is, especially the treatment before you go under and the treatment that you receive after the procedure. I felt the whole procedure was a wonderful experience. So, I talk to patients about my experience and tell them, "You don't have to worry, and you don't have to be that scared." I mean that it's a good thing.

Editor Commentary

It takes courage to create a completely new vision of an organization. It takes even more to announce that new vision to your community before you've achieved the results, but that's what the leadership of Sharp did when they shared The Sharp Experience with their employees, physicians, patients, and the entire San Diego regional community nearly simultaneously. It was a bold move and a different approach to branding than that used by most other healthcare systems.

Using the vision, driven throughout the organization by a committed senior leadership group, the onsite leaders have had the freedom and support to improve the patient experience and to engage their employees in making The Sharp Experience a reality everyday, even for endoscopy patients (not usually described as a "pleasant experience"). The passion for radically transforming the patient, staff, and physician experience is apparent in the Outpatient Pavillion leadership and has been translated into the performance of each individual staff member.

One particular aspect of how they created the "five-star model" stands out: the commitment to using—not just collecting—the data they have from patients, both quantitative and qualitative. They've also learned from best practices in other industries outside of healthcare, and they have made an upfront investment in education and training, especially with front-line employees. Employees were sent to observe other businesses, complete service maps, and establish the "ideal" patient experience. Next, employees were taught the expected behaviors and were videotaped in role-play situations, making the learning process experiential. It is rare that healthcare organizations make this type of up-front investment, and yet it seems integral to their success. Essentially, they have removed the "hope" factor—I "hope" these employees are "nice" to patients—by explicitly explaining and teaching what behaviors are expected. The employees are prepared to be overwhelmingly successful through practice, practice, and more practice. They completely set their employees up to be successful.

The enthusiasm the leaders and the staff have for their opportunity to excel comes through. Staff members clearly see and feel their connection to the entire patient/family experience and each other's daily work experience as well. The patient thank you cards and the enthusiasm they generate from both patients and the staff are but one example of this.

Leadership development and education have clearly played an important part of their ongoing success. Developing the individual leader's skill at employee selection and the subsequent emphasis on "the right fit" appear to be hallmarks of the organization. Leadership and personal accountability is apparent in the intolerance of unacceptable behaviors and of the willingness to coach employees along the right path. It also takes courage to "de-select" an employee; too many times managers just overlook nonperformance (and hope they get it eventually). The willingness to intervene is unusual.

Table 12-1   Organizational Demographics

Organization	Brigham and Women's Hospital, Member of Partners HealthCare System
Location	Boston, MA
Setting	Urban
Communities served	Urban and Suburban
Type of organization	Academic Medical Center
Number of beds	747
Number of FTEs	13,000
Scope of service	Brigham and Women's Hospital is a teaching affiliate of Harvard Medical School located in the heart of Boston's renowned Longwood Medical Area. Along with its modern inpatient facilities, BWH boasts extensive outpatient services and clinics, neighborhood primary care health centers, state-of-the-art diagnostic and treatment technologies, and research laboratories. BWH is a founding member of Partners HealthCare System, the largest integrated health care delivery network in New England. A top recipient of research grants from the National Institutes of Health—with an annual research budget of more than $400 million—BWH is internationally known for its clinical, translational, bench, and population-based research studies, including the landmark Nurses Health Study, Physicians Health Studies, and the Women's Health Initiative. In addition to being the regional leader in preeminent women's health services, BWH is also one of the nation's leading transplant centers, performing heart, lung, kidney, and heart–lung transplant surgery, as well as bone marrow transplantation. BWH is also nationally recognized for clinical and research excellence in cardiovascular medicine, neurosciences, arthritis and rheumatic disorders, orthopedics, and cancer care through the Dana-Farber/Brigham and Women's Cancer Center.
Organizational awards	National Quality Health Care Award; New England's Top Workplace for IT Professionals (given to Partners HealthCare System); ranked 11th on *U.S. News and World Report's* Honor Roll of America's Best Hospitals; inaugural Betsy Lehman Patient Safety Award; recognized by the University Health System Consortium for being one of the top three performing academic medical centers in the country in a special quality and safety benchmarking study
Focus area	Medical Residency Program
	The Brigham's internal medicine residency program is among the nation's most competitive and prestigious and has been the launching pad for numerous academic physician leaders. The tone of the program was initially established by the recently retired program director, whose leadership style has carried through to the current program leaders.

CHAPTER 12

Meritocracy

The stories in this chapter are the voices of the hospital CEO, the chief of medicine, the former and current directors of the medical residency program, former residents, attending physicians, current residents, administrative staff, stakeholders of the medical residency program, and nurses at Brigham & Women's Hospital. Here are their stories

BRIGHAM AND WOMEN'S HOSPITAL, MEMBER OF PARTNERS HEALTHCARE SYSTEM

Becoming a Doctor

Residency seems to me to be a series of challenges, and I typically have a lot of anxiety before one of the new challenges. It seems as you move from year to year there is always something new and more challenging that you are about to do. You are taking call for the first time. You are in the unit for the first time. You are the unit senior for the first time, and you run a code for the first time. Whatever it is, there is always a first time for something. For me, the satisfaction oftentimes comes at the end of the shift when I'm walking home or when I'm going to sleep for the night. I'll say, "I got through that day, and I feel like I did a pretty good job with it." For me, that's where satisfaction comes.

You just kind of have to jump through the hoops. As each successive experience builds on itself, you kind of gain confidence and feel a little bit better as you learn to recognize anxiety and say, "I understand I'm feeling incredibly anxious right now, but I also understand that I've felt this way for the last seven or eight exposures that I've had. I'll get through it and do fine." I think each time that eases a little bit. What the Brigham does well is surround you with resources. Even if you feel like you are on your own, you know that it's not hard to get help, and you're not really going to be looked down on for reaching out for that help. People at the Brigham care about the ultimate goal, which is to do the right thing for the patients we are taking care of.

I think it's that whole spirit of all pitching in and letting each person do his or her own thing. Also, they push the limits of what we are capable of doing and test that out. They allow interns to test out their ability to be a doctor, but not make it too hard for them to ask for help.

The whole goal of this program is to somehow take medical students and turn them into doctors. The senior people basically take a whole brand new group of medical students and start them on day 1 and guide them through the year, and at some point, the medical students become trained. When does that happen? How does that happen? When do you actually feel like a doctor?

In the beginning, you have no idea what you're doing. I think I realized that "wow, maybe I'm starting to get this" toward the end of my internship. The end of that first year of training is a transition time; the interns are about to become residents, and new interns arrive. That subordination relationship starts to shift. The residents are petrified because they are about to lose their trained interns and a new flock is about to come in. It's a very special time of the year.

The residents have the interns switch roles and "play" resident. The interns actually try to run rounds and try to prepare for what it will be like in just 20 days. So toward the end of my internship, I was playing resident and running rounds. I was on the oncology service, and we had an incredibly sick patient. No one knew exactly why he was sick or what was wrong with him. We were in this period of intensive diagnostic workup, and we essentially started from head to toe. I presented the case on rounds, and the resident looked at me and said, "Well, what do you want to do? You are running rounds."

I said, "This guy is incredibly sick. I have no idea where to start."

"Well," she said, "you're the resident."

The attending and I talked every day, and we went ahead and did a series of tests. Finally, it came down to the last test, a thoracentesis. I wanted to sample some pleural fluid. The resident didn't think we would find anything, but

I thought, "It's the only thing we haven't tested, and I wonder if the answer might be there." We did the thoracentesis and, in fact, made a diagnosis. It turned out to be a very interesting case. The patient had a treatable condition, and he did fine. So we had a celebration on rounds, and it was sort of like a send off.

The experience was affirming for me. It was the first time I took a case from the perspective of the doctor who decides what to do and how to approach it. It wasn't until someone said to me, "It's up to you—do what you want," that I started thinking, "Is there a risk to this procedure? How should I go about this?" It was a new and unique experience that made me realize, "Wow, I can take care of somebody. I can participate in a real way." That was sort of the first time I felt like a doctor. I think, if you are training to be a physician, that's got to be a peak. That's what you're here to do.

One satisfying moment I distinctly remember was very early in my junior year, at the end of my intern year. That year is all about feelings of being essentially inept and not able to master the challenges that everyone around you has already mastered. It's about being continuously reminded of your inability to really be a good doctor despite the fact that you came here to be one. Then you start junior year. This second year of training is the first time you are actually in a position of leadership and actually have new interns below you.

I remember being in the CCU one night as a newly minted junior resident. I realized that I actually had accrued some skills over one year, and it was a remarkable sort of confidence builder. While I couldn't necessarily articulate what those skills were, I realized that my pain and suffering as an intern paid off. You realize also that you draw from the support of your peers. There are those moments when you compare and trade notes with your colleagues and your peers. There are hallway exchanges in the morning when the postcall resident is leaving or when you drop off your bag and say, "I saw this really sick patient last night. Is there anything else I should have done?" When I think about that one very sick patient in July, it is a nice affirmation that I actually learned something. What a wonderful sort of experience that was.

I was a junior resident, and I was covering a patient who was unresponsive. The whole family was there, and they were very involved. I wanted to do a certain treatment, and they didn't agree with me. They said, "We want you to call the attending." It was maybe 11:30 at night, and I said, "This is what we need to do because he's really sick." They still didn't agree. So I called the attending who happened to be the past director of medical residency. He was in the emergency room at that time. He walked into the patient's room and said, "What's going on?"

So I told the story. He just said, "I completely agree," and walked out of the room, left, and went home. I felt like, "Whoa, he has confidence in my care of his patient." I think at that moment I truly felt like I was doing an okay job. That was a peak experience.

I was on the cardiac surgical rotation, and I had a patient who was supposed to have an aortic valve replacement. I was waiting for the patient to come out of the operating room because I was taught that you never go home until all of your patients are settled and stable. When the patient wasn't coming out, I got dressed in scrubs, and I went into the operating room. The patient was dying. His blood pressure was down. It wouldn't come up, and everyone was frustrated. The surgeon said that the patient's heart was like a baseball; it had frozen in a contracted state.

At that time, I knew there was a new drug that one of the cardiologists at the Brigham was using in a research study. It was a drug that made the heart and the blood vessels relax and dilate. I said to the surgeon, "Can I make a suggestion?"

He said, "At this point, I'll take advice from anyone."

So I told him there was a new drug we might try. He told me to go ahead and get it. I ran downstairs and found the cardiologist, and we found a few capsules of this drug. We carried them upstairs, poked holes in them, and squirted the capsules in the patient's mouth. The patient's heart relaxed, filled with blood, and his blood pressure came up. He was fine. For a minute I just sort of sat there.

That night I said to my friend, "I just want to watch this guy breathe." When you actually save a patient's life, there's nothing that compares, but the patient would have died if not for the Brigham environment: the research going on and the high clinical standards we have. It would not have happened if we weren't conducting a research study on this drug, if I hadn't been taught to stay with my patients until they are stable, and if the surgeon hadn't been willing to take advice from a young trainee.

One of my peak experiences was after my first time as a code leader. A code blue requires a huge interdisciplinary approach: an anesthesiologist, nurses, interns, residents, and a whole team of like 12 people trying to stabilize the patient. I distinctly remember being an intern and being deathly afraid of codes and wanting to go to a different floor when a code was called. So as a third-year medicine resident and code leader who had basically just watched this chaotic situation in the past, I realized that suddenly somehow after three years I knew what to do. Now when a code happens I actually run toward it, and I actually really enjoy running them because it's clinically interesting; it requires a huge team effort, and it's satisfying to stabilize some of these very sick patients. It was a real mark for me in terms of how far I've come.

There was an episode where a patient I was taking care of had a disease called atrial fibrillation. The patient was on a blood thinner, and on admission to the hospital, the levels on the blood thinner were too low. The patient needed to have a procedure done, and we were trying to decide when to restart the blood thinner safely after the procedure. As a consequence of the abnormal blood thinner levels, the patient unfortunately had a stroke. I was devastated, really upset about the event. The patient's stroke ended up being a rather mild stroke, but nonetheless, it felt horrible having interviewed the patient, worked with the patient, cared for him, and then watch him go through this. It was heartbreaking. In those moments, my boss validated my care, my emotions, and my angst in a professional and appropriate manner. It made it feel okay, and it helped me understand those responsibilities, problems, and difficulties in taking care of patients. I remember he took that valley and turned it into a moment that I've always remembered. He likes to say that the art of medicine is making difficult decisions with an incomplete database. One doesn't always have science to guide you. That was one of those times. So I think that even though it was difficult it was a really memorable experience. It helps me when I interact with patients on a daily basis, even today.

When you have a very complicated case, a patient who you are really scratching your head about and you don't really understand what's going on, this is the kind of place where intellectual curiosity is allowed to run free. At the Brigham, you really have the ability to mobilize resources and get consultants and get a lot of people on board and do unusual things that you wouldn't even necessarily think about in a typical medical setting. We have the ability to go beyond the hospital floor and try to mobilize resources in the laboratory and other clinical settings and to seek help from other institutions to try to figure out what's going on with the patient. It is most rewarding when that does happen and you have the opportunity to go beyond what you might consider routine medical care and actually figure out what's going on with the patient.

I always make sure that I am attending on the medicine service in July when the new residents come in. It's an intensive period where I'm right there on the floor taking care of the patients with the new interns and residents. There is one particular example I remember when a young woman who had many chronic medical problems was admitted to the hospital. She and her daughters decided that they didn't want to fight it anymore. This was it. They wanted to back off on care. This is an emotionally difficult decision for a family and for a physician. In this situation, the physician had only been a physician for two weeks. So I had this group of interns meet with the family, and we spent a lot of time at the bedside with the patient. I kind of walked that particular physician through the process, and we talked about the family's fears and the issues that this brought up for the patient. In the end, the family wrote a letter saying they were very grateful for how things worked out. The intern also expressed his gratitude for having had the opportunity to learn about this incredibly challenging time at a very threatening part of his own career. All physicians want their patients to do well, especially when they are brand new interns. I think that this is the type of valuable learning experience that we try to provide our trainees.

Most doctors in training don't really get a chance to spend any durable quality time with the patient and understand exactly what their illness becomes during treatment. When I was in training, patients were admitted for two weeks if they had heart failure. By the end of the two-week period, I knew exactly what was going to happen after they got treated, and I knew exactly what to predict. The next time I saw a patient with heart failure it was pretty straightforward.

That is not the case now. Patients have much shorter hospital stays and then are discharged or they go to another team, and they leave the residency training program. The experiential view of how to train as a resident and what to learn from their training is quite different than it used to be.

I use that as an example of what is missing in our current traditional training environment. Patients have to be discharged so quickly that there is no way for a physician to know exactly what the benefits or failings of his or her treatment might be. I pointed out that the Brigham ought to take a lead in redesigning how residents are trained and that I would be happy to lead the process. I suggested that the hospital should support it because having better trained residents means the place has a better reputation, has better outcomes, saves money, and improves quality. It's a win for everybody; it's a modest investment for that win.

Selection

We have three selection criteria. The first one is clinical excellence. You have to be very smart, top of your class, and clinically devoted. Criteria number two, and this is where I think we're very fortunate, we prioritize interpersonal skills. There are a lot of bright people in the world, but we actually have built a system that allows us to pick the people who are bright and nice. The third criterion is that we look for people who want to make a difference and people who have a vision. We are not particular or restrictive about what that vision is. We have a lot of graduates who have gone on to be great scientists, but we are equally proud of our graduates who contribute to community health, international medicine, health policy, or medical education. It's sort of that spark in the applicant's eyes that says, "I'm not going to be content until I've improved that delivery of care in some way." Those are our three criteria. I think you can have those goals in any organization, but you have to be able to back them up with the allocation of resources in order to perpetuate it.

Every year we have the challenge and the opportunity to recruit and sign up 68 new doctors. Every July we review the applications from around the country, and we invite about 10% of those for interviews. We have a very frank meeting where we tell them what our mission is. We say, "Things will change, but the mission is not going to change. If you are not interested in that mission or if it doesn't excite you, then you are probably better off somewhere else. If on the other hand, that's what you are looking for, that's what you are going to get here."

When they interview people for the program, one of the things they look for in addition to clinical excellence is interpersonal skills. That is actually one of the criteria, and that really surprised me when I heard it.

My interview for the residency program, I still remember, was exactly seven minutes long. Most of these interviews run at least like 30 to 40 minutes. He asked me about four questions, did not give me time to finish any of the answers, and then announced almost immediately, "I'm done here. If you have anything else to say, feel free to ask. Otherwise, I think we can wrap this up." I figured I was cooked. I walked out a little shell shocked, but then I saw a senior resident who said, "My interview was short too, and I'm here. That's what happens." They know what they are looking for, get the information that they need, and then get out.

I thought I wanted to be a cardiologist at the time, and this was by far the most premier institution for cardiology. So in my interview with a residency leader I was asked, "So you want to be a cardiologist?"

I said, "Yeah, I think so."

"Why?"

"Well, I really enjoy it."

"Okay."

"Anyhow, we really need a cellist here."

I'm a musician, and I actually spend a lot of time playing music.

The physician leader said, "We could use a cellist." Essentially, he was saying we have nine cardiologists, but you have another quality. The Brigham was a place that really seemed to have a sense of who you were when you walked in the door. Despite the 30-second interview, the physician leader has this unique way of dropping hints along the way that he actually is paying attention. He actually really does know who you are. Somehow, despite the trillions of people he manages, he catalogs something about each person. That's his connection with you.

Ironically, I interviewed at another place, and they wanted to know why I wasn't coming. For me it was a no-brainer. One place was nurturing, and one was stiff, formal, and hierarchal. There was no question in my mind.

I think we can appreciate that it is the program's advocacy for the residents that is really remarkable. The leaders in the residency program are amazing assessors of character. Everyone has great stories about selecting people with great speed and accuracy. Time and again they have picked ranks of residents who are motivated, who are bright, and who are also fun to train with.

Which personal qualities am I looking for in my trainees? Well, just to even be considered, you have to be academically gifted and accomplished. Beyond that, we look for people who pass the Sandbox Test, which is to say that they work and play well with others. Then finally, we hope that the people who come here will some day be contributors and will make us proud. Now, we don't care necessarily about the arena in which they contribute. It may be patient care. It may be teaching. It may be research, but we would like to think that the people who come here will add value back to society, and they do.

When people come to our program, they are always impressed that we have the nicest, happiest, most nurturing residents of any place they've visited.

They ask, "How do you do that?" We tell them it's our selection process that's unique.

I feel very proud of having created a program where we value people's personal qualities and their interactive skills and style as much as their academic achievements. I feel proud of having set up a system where we use house staff on the selection committee. Every year at the internship committee I get up and say, "I think it's very important to remember that we are picking people we want to work with and not just people who we want on the faculty to write papers." That value remains and is somewhat unique to the program. It is one of the things that makes our program distinct.

Our approach is very unadorned. Here's what you get. This is not the time for a fancy slide show about our big operation, how much money we have, and all of the programs available. Instead, we take a very unadorned philosophy that it's not the bricks and mortar that count—it's the mission that counts. The simpler and more direct you can be, the better.

Meritocracy

Medicine can be a very hierarchal system; it has traditionally been so. The Brigham blew that out of the water. Interns are our colleagues, our future colleagues. We are here to train them because they are part of us. We do not abuse them; they are not here to do our scut work. The whole aura of how we deal with our colleagues is not "how can we destroy the people beneath us to make our way up." Instead, we think of it as "this is our future; this is what we invest in."

"Interns take care of patients, and residents take care of interns." That pretty much sums it up. There was never an expectation that you would reach a level of entitlement in the program and then just go off and do your own thing.

The goal of the medical residency program is to create leaders as opposed to worker bees. There are many kinds of leaders. There are leaders as clinicians, leaders as teachers, and leaders as scientists. I think that the mixture among these three categories of leaders changes from year to year, but we are looking for people who are going to be at the top.

A value that perhaps is a bit more unique is that we pride collegiality above almost all things. We try very hard when screening applicants to find and select students not only based on their academic excellence or extracurricular activities or so forth, but really on personality. We want to assemble a diverse group of people who have a wide range of interests so that we can create a very diverse and heterogeneous hospital and also people who have wonderful personalities to make it simply a great place to work. It's wonderful to be surrounded by, in my case in my class, 60 residents. I know that all of them are ready to back me up at the drop of a hat if I need help.

At the Brigham, calling the resident is not a sign of weakness at all. You are expected to. You work together all night long. I really liked that, and I tried to do that for my own interns when I became a resident and then also as an attending. When I started the Women's Health Center at the Brigham I tried very much to make it a nonhierarchal group. We all learned from each other: nurses, physicians, and staff. One of the best compliments I got was from the chief of OB/GYN who told me that he thought my practice was unique. The patients were happy. The doctors were happy, and the staff was happy. He said that in most practices you get two out of three, but he had never seen three out of three. I think that makes a really effective team. Everyone has a say, whether it's the nurses or the health assistants. Everybody can bring something to the table, and it's up for discussion.

I was on oncology, and we were done for the day; my resident was ready to go home. A nurse approached me and said, "There's a family member who wants to speak with you." So I went up to see this patient who had come in with a new diagnosis of leukemia. I went in to see him, and his daughter said, "My dad, he is just in this weird sleep." I knew enough to realize that that wasn't just sleep. The patient was vegetative but still had a heartbeat. I was freaked out. I must have had the look of death on my face because a resident who was nearby said, "Are you okay?"

I said, "No." It was my first experience ever really seeing somebody dying. I had no one there really from my team. That resident didn't go home but instead mobilized everything that needed to get done to stabilize the patient and move him to the ICU. She took me through the whole transfer of this patient even though it wasn't her patient. She wasn't on the team, and she wasn't even on call. Then I got to the ICU, and another colleague, who wasn't on call, assisted me. Everybody was there until about 10:00 at night.

Afterward, I was still there ruminating over this patient and trying to deal with how this had happened, and I felt pretty terrible. Then I got a page, out of the blue, from a friend of mine who said, "I just heard about what happened." She wasn't on call either. Basically, three residents who weren't even responsible for that patient or me were there in the late hours of the night helping me through it. It was more for me than the patient. That's when I realized the program was something pretty unique. That would never have happened anywhere else.

After I graduated from medical school, when I considered where to go to train, it was Boston, Boston, Boston. I interviewed all over town, but the Brigham made a big impression on me. This was a training program where I would be with colleagues and other trainees who all were like-minded in thought. They were smart. They were inquisitive. They were relaxed, and they were not supercompetitive. There was a comfort around that.

I think that people take enormous pride in this organization. It's not just a place where you have a job. If something bad happens, everybody is upset, like a family would be. If something good happens, it's everybody's joy. It is very different than coming from an office where there is very little association, where you are looking for a paycheck, and maybe make improvements so that you can take it somewhere else. Many of the people at the Brigham, the physicians and nurses, make this a destination job, as opposed to a transient thing. There is a high level of commitment to personal quality of work because people around you are very good; therefore, you don't want to be less than the others.

Even though I was doing unconventional things, I got very good academic advice. I was able to get grants and write papers and ultimately become a professor. I got nothing but support as I took a conventional approach to unconventional areas. Over time, I moved into management. Today I'm one of the senior management at Partners in Healthcare, and I continue to get support. The leaders of the residency program had more imagination about what I could do than I did. I came here because it was a meritocracy, but it turned out to be a much more creative, nurturing environment than I could have anticipated.

I think the major thing that makes this place special is it is a true meritocracy. We really believe in that, and we have tried to enable people to identify their own paths and then to pursue their dreams, with vigor and support from the organization.

Fierce Loyalty

I love the Brigham, and I would do anything they would ever ask me to do. They have been very good to me.

The Brigham has a philosophy unlike some of the other teaching hospitals around. They really do take care of their own and are very family oriented. I think they do more here to take care of family members of the staff.

I picked this place because I thought the program director was so dedicated to the residents and not afraid to stand up to the hospital administration or anyone else to make sure the residents got the best quality education.

I remember thinking as a medical student that everybody wanted to come here and everybody had this awe-like view of what it was like. It is not easy to be an intern or a resident, but everyone here seemed sort of part of a family no matter how bad things were going.

The people within the program really take care of each other. Attending physicians are important, but the people who really teach you are the residents you work with every day. What was transmitted to me is that everyone within the system knows each other and looks out for each other. So on a day-to-day basis, if you go to someone and say I need help, people will drop what they're doing to help you. Similarly, if you tell the leadership that you need help, it will happen. It may be a very brief encounter; you may have no idea what transpired, but days later you will get whatever it was that you asked for—almost uniformly. I think the legend of this program is not only to recruit talented, smart people, but also to take care of them once they are here. I think it is unusual to the degree that it happens here, within a Harvard institute.

I pinch myself every morning thinking how lucky I am to work with the people here. They are committed to excellence, but also committed to taking care of each other.

Enduring Relationships

I guess if I could wave a magic wand it would be that the people I train with could actually stay together and work together for the rest of our careers. We are a great group, and we have formed wonderful relationships. We may not make relationships like this again.

When I came up here to interview, it was pretty clear that the Brigham stood apart in terms of the camaraderie with the house staff.

The camaraderie among the residents brings life to the department. We have little gatherings, whether it is a Halloween party or holiday party. Not only do we get the residents involved, but we also invite their families and their children. We cater to the core family rather than just to the employee, and that shows concern for the person not just the worker.

I think there is a gigantic sense of camaraderie and spirit here because we are all in it together—going through unique experiences that we haven't been through before. We make new core friendships that will continue onward. Most of my closest friends in Boston are people who I was a co-resident with. The things we went through the hard times, your first patient dying, things going poorly, making mistakes, and also the great times when things go well—are a big part of it. There is a general emphasis on people having a good quality of life in the residency program and people make sure that if you work hard you play hard, and if you are here a lot, then you go out and have a life outside of the hospital. I think this place encourages you to have a life outside of the hospital, which is important.

When I was an intern, in my first night on call, there was a patient who got really sick. I was really quite upset because I had formed a good relationship with this patient. At the time I felt like, "Oh, could I have changed the outcome?" I remember the resident on the service that day said, "You know what? You are too upset." That night she called her husband, and they took me out for dinner. For hours we sat there talking about death and getting close to patients. I remember they talked to me until I felt better and more confident. It was sort of my lowest point and maybe my highest point because it made me realize how wonderful the residents are here and the sense of family.

I've maintained a mentoring relationship with many of the people I've trained. One person who left the country came back a couple of times over the last year. It was clear that although he was very pleased with his job, his wife was deriving less satisfaction out of her position in Geneva. Every time he came to Boston he'd come by to see me. I told him, "Come back. We'll find your wife a good job." He always maintained his relationship with the department, and through negotiations and support from a lot of people who were very anxious to see him come back, we managed to convince him to come back to America and to us. That was a great triumph for our program.

Everyone I knew who had any sort of contact with the Brigham, at any station in their career, all raved about the place and said what a wonderful experience it was. In particular, everyone pointed out how wonderful the people were. It's not just one person or two people, but a dozen people who were all telling me the same thing. That really means that there is something special about the place, and that's what really attracted me to even consider this place.

Dedication to Patients

Helping patients and the people who are tending to the patients definitely brings me here every day. I make sure the intern's needs are met so that they can do the job that they need to do.

We take good care of patients, too. I think it's worth mentioning that as focused as we are about our own training, there is emphasis on patient care.

We have a mission here of always putting our patients first. A lot of that stems from the past director of medical residency because he is such a great clinician. We all respect him, and we all want to be a little bit like him in the way we take care of patients. So I think we try to go that extra mile for our patients, sort of something we've learned here, and we carry it forward.

We contribute to the high satisfaction scores in our organization by staying out of people's way. I think that we strive to make a culture where people who work here are empowered to make it better for themselves and for those that follow.

I think the culture of the department of medicine is one in which you don't go home until you've taken care of your patients. We never actually sign our beepers out unless we are out of the country. The culture that I was raised with when I was a house officer was to be very fiercely dedicated to your patients and never sign things over to other people . . . ever.

I don't like the phrase "ownership of patients" because I don't think that sounds right. Ultimate responsibility for the care of the patient is the spirit that's engendered here from the very beginning. There are so many instances where I've seen that. I've had interns whose patients had multiple studies that needed to be done. Normally you could sign out to another person to check up on the patient, but they stayed to find out the results themselves and also gave the results to the patient. That is not the exception; it is relatively common.

I think we try to make our patients happy. Don't get me wrong, but I don't think that is the highest value and goal we have. Patient satisfaction here probably comes more so from individual experiences, and I think that just flows from the fact that there are pretty good-hearted people here. People don't really go about bragging or trumpeting themselves about those experiences. I was just reading the newsletter the other day about someone who brought an MP3 player with soothing music and put it by the patient's bedside. The patient actually ended up nominating her for the Starfish Award, which has to do with excellence. The thing is, I know her, and she would never have told anyone that story.

I can think of one particular instance where I had a very powerful experience with a patient who came in while I was on vacation. She was a young person with a disease that she eventually died from. I came in to see her when I wasn't on service and made the effort to get to know her and her family. We make that kind of commitment to our patients by going above and beyond to make a connection. As chief resident, I definitely saw multiple residents have those kind of relationships with patients, relationships where they really invest in the person, not just the patient. They got to know that person and would come back at the end of the day to sit and talk or made time on the weekends to come in and see a patient when they didn't need to. There are certainly many residents who have gone to patients' homes to visit them.

A particular patient was dying. It was the last few days of his life, and I was working all of those days in a row. At a certain point in this situation, the relationship is not really with the patient anymore, because they are not talking, but with their family.

This patient just one day all of a sudden said, "I don't want to do this anymore. I've had enough, and I want to go home." We worked so hard as a team, the resident, the social worker, the patient's family, and me, just trying to get that patient home. I think it must have taken the resident five hours that morning, as though he had no other patients.

It came to be that the patient was getting so sick that we didn't think it was a smart idea to send him home. The resident was afraid the patient would die in the ambulance with only his wife there. So the resident called in all of the family members. They all were there. When the patient actually passed away, everyone was there. We sat with the family, and while the patient passed away, we were able to look at him as a person, beyond the crisis.

I remember a story that has to do with accountability and responsibility. Christmas time for interns is a particularly difficult time. As an intern we were on call every other night over a six-day stretch around the Christmas holiday. On Christmas Eve, there was a patient—I still remember exactly what room she was in and which bed she was in. It's one of those haunting images that will stay with me forever. The patient had an extremely aggressive lung cancer. She was obviously doing poorly; it was unlikely she would survive this. Regardless, we wondered how long we could keep her alive. The only thing that the family wanted was that she not die on Christmas Day.

The attending, who previously didn't know this patient, came by and was rounding with me. We had to launch into the discussion with the patient and the family about what her long-term wishes were, how she wanted to be treated if she would need to go on a breathing machine. It was incredibly awful and horrible to have the discussion anytime, much less around the time of the holidays. It was ultimately decided that if she were to get sicker she would not go to the ICU, but we would do everything possible to take care of her on the floor.

I actually sat at her bedside on Christmas day, and we administered chemotherapy with an oncology nurse who came down from the floor. The care coordinator worked all morning long to arrange hospice. Throughout the day, the patient seemed to settle out. It looked like she would make it through the night. They were actually having a Christmas day dinner on the floor at the nursing station. When she stopped breathing, everybody ran in the room. It was this sort of surreal mix of a party going on with this woman dying in front of us on Christmas day. We tried everything possible, short of putting her on a ventilator, but unfortunately, she died. So I had to call the family.

It is now 11:00 at night on Christmas day, and the attending who had rounded with me earlier actually came in. All of us were standing there with the family at midnight on Christmas. They were obviously devastated, but they essentially turned to us and said, "We understand. You did everything you could, and we are incredibly grateful." At the same time, I was pretty amazed that the attending, who didn't even know this person, had mobilized all of the stuff to happen and came back in when the patient died. This shows how we are ownership driven to the point where we say, "Look. I'll be right there. It's Christmas day, but I'm coming in."

We have a program where we encourage residents to do home visits, and they have been extremely successful. I always tell my residents about my experiences with home visits. One time when I made a home visit, it was just so successful that it inspired me to do more. On one occasion, I had to cancel my clinic because I had to give a talk or something. I heard from the clinic that the patient's daughter was very disappointed because I canceled. I was very close to this patient, and I was so upset to disappoint her. She was overweight, had high blood pressure, and was taking care of her husband who had a stroke. I called the patient back, and I told her, "You know what? I'm going to come visit you at your house because I couldn't see you in the office. Is that okay?"

I was always encouraging her to take her medications, and she would say, "Yeah, I'm so busy taking care of my husband that sometimes I don't do such a good job taking care of myself." So when I got to her home, she had laid out this little spread for me, nice little treats and everything, and her house was just so spic and span, so nice. It was just great to see the whole setup. Her husband, who had a stroke but could still communicate, pointed to all of his medications that she's laid out for him. Then he pointed to her medications that she often doesn't take. Then he took me downstairs and showed me this beautiful treadmill he bought for her with an armchair there next to it. I said, "My goodness. Why aren't you coming down here to exercise? Your husband can sit right next to you." The husband was nodding his head. He pointed to a TV he put down there for her. Later, whenever I would see her, I would always tell her, "Look what your husband did for you. You should be exercising," and she would laugh.

It was just kind of interesting to see that model of family life; it was fantastic. I always tell my residents about this. It completely changed how I looked at her. When you see patients in the hospital wearing a Johnny, you really don't have a sense of who they really are. When you see them in the office, they are all dressed up, and you have a better sense. When you see them in their home, with all of their possessions around them, their family photos and what's important to them, it just makes a huge difference. I love this program about the residents going to a home. They all love it, and that really does lead to great patient satisfaction.

There is a woman, who was a Brigham resident, who is the most caring person I've ever met. She takes care of patients who are HIV positive and really, really poor. When these patients would leave her office, she always hugged them, and they always kissed her because they really loved her. Her office was right across from mine, and I would hear her talking to her patients, and she would say, "You know. You really need to be doing this or that." She would say, "Look, as your doctor and I hope your friend, I am telling you that you really need to be doing this." It influenced me so much because I felt that why not hug your patients? I think it makes them feel so connected. Why hold back from that? I learned a great deal from her, and she always made home visits. In fact, one time, one of her patients, who was blind and used a walker, was evicted from his apartment. She got out and went into her car and drove around the neighborhood to look for him.

I do think it's a privilege to be a doctor, and it's a privilege to have people entrust their care to me. I try to take that very seriously, and I focus on every patient individually and give him or her my best. I hope I am successful. If I'm not, I am certainly trying all the time, and it's not just about taking care of patients in the office. Even when I'm not with them I think about their problems and try to come up with solutions by talking to others. I think it's really an honor to be entrusted with this privilege and the big responsibility that goes with it.

Blame-Free Culture

We have done a lot of work to get the board engaged in the whole quality effort. There is a board committee called the Care Improvement Council. It is kind of the quality committee of the hospital, and it passes on appointments and has to review cause analyses. I made the decision pretty early that the biggest fiduciary responsibility or risk that a board member has here is really related to safety and quality, greater than to finances. I was very emphatic with the chair of the board that this was a huge fiduciary responsibility. We present stuff to them that's scary. We want them to understand the specifics of a particular case, what the risks are, what human error is, and what we are doing structurally to eradicate that. We want them to see how we implement things and what the follow-up is, and they are truly engaged in it. The amount of time that he commits to us, and the value that we get from his brain, as well as his time, is commendable.

There is a warm and nurturing learning environment here. If I made a mistake, I wouldn't be a pariah. I would learn from it, and patients would get better care because I learned more quickly.

No matter what, life is about making mistakes, learning about mistakes, and then next time making a different choice.

In terms of the blame, here it is not punitive. It's looked at as a system error. What failed in the system?

Our whole philosophy has changed. We don't call them "incident reports" because that had more of a punitive spin to it. We call it "safety reporting." That's what it's about: It's about safety.

Errors are viewed as foundational. We do the safety reporting sheets as a review, but if a mistake is made, whether it's per nursing or whether it's house staff, as a team they go into the room and they address this to the patient. "It seems as though there was an error made. We apologize for it." So actually they are telling you to go in and tell them, apologize, which is a whole different mindset than I think existed in the past.

There was a patient on the surgical service who did not have the best outcome. One of my colleagues went to visit the patient every day, and because it was a changing of service, she sort of took the ball and really helped him coordinate his care so that he would get the care that he needed. She also worked with the hospital to help finance the extra care that he needed at home. The family was so grateful to her. They said she was the only person who had really showed an interest in them and really helped them with their day-to-day details. This woman had really taken charge of every detail. It made such a huge impression on me. Sometimes when things go wrong, if it's not directly your fault, it's hard to step in, take responsibility, and say, "I'm really sorry that things didn't go your way." I think that's a really hard thing to do, and I was impressed by her in this situation for doing that.

The hospital has been extremely full. This hospital budgets around 89% occupancy; about 85% occupancy is homeostasis for a general medical center to operate. That occupancy is at midnight, which means during the day it's more than that. Over the course of the last couple of weeks we've had more than the capacity of the hospital with people waiting in the emergency room, no beds available.

We made walk rounds. We tried to probe for what kinds of things people saw, and people kept saying everything was perfect. We take very detailed minutes of those walk rounds and then get back to the team immediately after we summarized it. We have a six-month closing cycle where we try to close every item, and I think we have an 80% close rate, which is good, given how broad some of the things people ask for—it's hard to build a parking lot in a week. So I started to talk about the "business" of the hospital, the relationship between the floor and the emergency room, and the various issues of communication. People started to talk about the interaction between the order entry systems, a lack of knowledge of who was on call, and who was responsible for the patient. I pushed harder, and people provided a variety of details that could help us to repair the situation.

I saw a medical resident who was actually entering orders at a workstation, and I could see her responding emotionally to some comment that was made. So I engaged her and asked her what was going on. She said that she had been on call the day before, and she couldn't access one of the patients she had admitted. This was a barrier. She described the problem in great detail, and we got back to her as to how we could fix this situation. We actually changed something within an hour of that meeting in terms of entry, access, and information flow.

Traditions

Our emphasis is on really bringing the best and the brightest people together to care for the sickest and neediest populations, reaching out to our community, and making that commitment in a real way. There is a commitment to teaching the next generation of future leaders, which is a critical component of what we do.

Each December and January when we invite our potential new doctors. We have a one- or two-day program for the candidates. This is a big group, and we spend the first hour going around from person to person. We have studied their charts prior to this so that we know them in detail. As we go around, we are trying to remember who was the bike rider, who was the chef, etc. We were trying to keep those things together. We try to make every introduction personal. For example, I might say, "Hey, John. How are you? It's fantastic that you pitched for the Durham Bulldogs. That's amazing."

They'll say, "How did you know that?"

Or we'll say, "I really enjoyed the letter that was written by Dr. so and so. He and I worked together when we were at the NIH." We try to make every conversation personal.

As an intern my first year, I had a really hard year. I knew that I had done the job, but I had no idea whether I did a good job or not. I got a little handwritten note card in the mail from the director. It was maybe five sentences that basically said that I had done a great job, that he felt privileged to work with me, and that he hoped that I would consider being one of his chief residents in the future. I was just blown away. I had no idea. It made me feel special. It made me feel great about the job I had done. It made me come back really motivated to do another great job the next year. While I don't promise people that they are going to be chief residents, I now try to send people a handwritten note card to tell them thank you for doing such a good job.

A group of residents noticed that the nurses were working incredibly hard to take care of a patient. They were going way above and beyond the call of duty, but there was no real formal recognition from the house staff of the nurses' efforts. Of course, there was always that immediate kind of thank you, such a great job, but there was no real way of saying in public, "You're a special person, and you've done a special job with your patient." So we put together a nursing recognition award that was given by the department of medicine and the house staff for nurses who had really gone above and beyond the call of duty. We worked with nursing leadership. The house staff identified the nurses that they wanted to honor, and we asked nursing leadership to coordinate that process. They set up a day where we had nurses come together, and we announced the winners. The first time we did this I was blown away. We did it at lunch one day during nursing week in the spring. The nurses came, and their significant others came. Their kids came, and their friends came. In a room where we expected to have maybe 40 to 50 people, there were like 200 people. It was awe inspiring. The house staff got up and told a little anecdote about each of the award winners and then announced their name. The recognition came directly from house staff to the nurse. We continue to do this each year. It was a wonderful event where everybody was really moved. It has led to improved communication and interaction between the house staff and the nursing staff as well.

A young person in my program had a patient here, and the patient got transferred to another hospital into hospice care. He was dying. On this young man's night off, he would bike to the other hospital to see this patient. The patient was no longer on service here, and the intern was already working 100 hours a week; however, he would go up there two, three, four nights a week to be with that patient and his family. The family was so grateful. They said, "We want to do something to recognize this person. What would be a good way to do this?" I think they really thought they should give this person a gift. I told them I thought it would be nice to recognize his spirit. So we set up an award, really in his honor, that the family funded. It is a recognition award for interns who go above and beyond the usual norm in caring for their patients. Often a member of that family will come, and the young man who rode his bicycle would actually do the presentation. He is now a senior member of the faculty, and I still see him in a mentorship role. It's really very rewarding.

I got an incredible letter from the son of one of our patients who wrote this really very touching and beautiful letter about one particular intern who made such an impact on their lives. The intern was so caring and thoughtful and even after the father was discharged called home to make sure that all the medications were going well. I sent it back to the letter writer, and I thanked him very much for writing the letter. Then I copied the usual suspects, the president of the hospital, the department chairman, our educational faculty, the chief residents, and the intern. I said, "Thank you for making us look good, but more importantly, thank you for your outstanding contributions to patient care," and I quoted it in his fellowship letter as well. I received a similar letter when I was an intern, and it buoyed me up. Now I try to carry that tradition on.

I used to make house calls to a patient because it was hard for him to come see me. He would always get very upset because Medicare would pay me about $18 to $20 to spend an hour with him on Sunday, and he thought that was not adequate compensation for my time. I would say to him, "It's all right. Some day you are going to give me a bunch of money for the house staff."

He has since set up two funds, which have grown through the years, and now generate sufficient support for two instructors in the department. I can now fund people who want to do projects or fund people who want to do educational things, and it has been very important to our department. As it happens, he was the beginning of a whole group of extraordinarily generous people who have supported our program. One of the things that allows us to do very innovative things is we have a lot of resources that most programs don't have.

I just saw patients this morning, and I'm still seeing patients in the teaching clinic, as I have since 1979. Some of the patients I've followed for well over two decades—many of them are quite rich, but many of them are quite poor. So the mission of never turning anyone away for lack of resources is a core part of the identity that makes people like me very proud to have been part of the Brigham.

Another interesting tradition that began with the opening of the hospital was that was the chief of medicine basically selected the next chief of surgery, and the next chief of surgery selected the next chief of medicine. So, therefore, that created some bond. I was selected by the chief of surgery, and when he retired, I selected his successor, and that person selected mine.

As a result, there is a very good relationship between people in the department of medicine and the department of surgery. Those departments are usually quite competitive. There are often turf battles between medicine and surgery, battles over patients and philosophical battles about approaching the patients, and ultimately, it does have something to do with income; however, I was amazed when I came here that I didn't sense that at all. That's one of the things that struck me as different.

Nurturing Others

There is a Quaker adage that says you should always look for the inner light within every person. I try to do that. I don't try to tell people what they should be. I try to help them identify what it is that excites them and help them get there.

My mission is to attract the most talented, young physicians to train here and then to nurture them so that they achieve their potential.

A core value we have is to provide outstanding training and flexibility that allows trainees to become both great doctors and great leaders in their own field. I think you can be inflexible and become a great doctor. I think it's hard to become a great leader unless you are given the opportunities to go in your own direction, and that's where we pride ourselves.

There is no mission statement that is really associated with our program, but having been here long enough, I think the philosophy of the program is that whatever it is you want to do, they want to help you develop to become that. There is no constraint. There is no pigeonholing. There is no saying, "Well, you're going to be a basic scientist. You're going to be an epidemiologist, or this is what you should do." Instead, it's really self-driven. When you say, "This is what I want to do," the residency program makes it possible. There is enormous flexibility. If there are unusual things you want to do, even outside the traditional medical scale, they make it possible. They allow you to take time off and go to other countries or go to labs really anywhere in the country or the world. They will make that happen. I think their mission is to help us develop to be whatever it is that we want to be.

The people who graduate from here are definitely leaders in their field, especially in nontraditional areas. We definitely have a famous cardiology program. We have world-class oncologists, but what I really appreciate is that many of my internists are somewhat nontraditional. I felt like I could have a home here at the Brigham and be nurtured, mentored, and supported in the same way as someone with more traditional academic and clinical medicine aspirations.

I think the number one is definitely the people. They have supported me and allowed me to test out different things. My interest is in medical education, and the Brigham affords me the chance to test out novel ideas in medical education and gives me an awesome environment for trying those things out.

There is great flexibility from the organization in allowing us to participate in the varied activities required for innovation. There is no blueprint that directs you to go the straight and narrow. They really have been very understanding of people who want to do things a different way. It's a really unique environment here at the Brigham.

A lot of people have gone on to do great things from our program, but one that I feel especially proud was 10 to 15 years ago two very bright, talented, and accomplished young people were applying for the program, and they were very interested in improving the healthcare of the underserved. They started in medical school to take a very active role in an area of Haiti that didn't have very good health resources. They decided to see if they could develop resources for that population. They were about to go on an internship, which is usually a full-time job, and I created a way for them to alternate between time here and in Haiti. So one of them would be here, and one would be in Haiti. From time to time, when they faced financial crises, I would help them there, too. I think that the ability to support them financially as well as the flexibility of the program is important.

We permitted them to pursue this activity throughout the course of their training by creating a somewhat unique program for them, and today they run Partners in Health. One of them has just returned from being the Deputy Director of the World Health Organization, now head of our Social Medicine.

There is a plan to have an even more international focus of the residency program. We have a program at the Brigham, the division of social medicine, where people can do their internship at the Brigham, and then I think part of the residency is overseas. You go to resource-poor locations, and you sort of really learn how to deliver high-quality care with very few resources.

I meet with the group of residents each week for an hour, and I really enjoy that session because it gives me the opportunity to talk not so much about medicine, but to talk about administrative issues in a creative way. Half of their job is administrative, as they become leaders among the house staff. They deal with a lot of leadership challenges. For example, they were concerned about the way the cardiology teams had been organized. They were worried that the balance of the house staff experience was not optimal when they rotated on these two cardiology services. One was very busy. One was less so. One was highly specialized. One was less so, and they wanted to think about a way to change that. So we talked about changing the process. We came up with a strategy about how they can reach a consensus and which would be the most influential of these groups of people. They did a great job, and I think things are going to change for the better.

One of the wonderful things about working with the leadership in this program is that they didn't just know I was married—he knew my wife's name and my kids' names. So there was an attention to that personal detail that I didn't expect. It was very important to my training and career development.

Most recently, when I was on the medical service, there was a patient who had a less than desirable outcome. We, as a team, brought everybody together, and we just sat and talked with the family. We felt we owed the husband an explanation for exactly what had happened and also an apology. I had recently attended a panel discussion lead by a surgeon who was very interested in medical error. At that conference, he had emphasized the power of apology. He said that when you make a mistake it's important to apologize, to say that it was your fault, to show empathy, and to make amends.

It was really interesting leading the team through that. I was using this opportunity to teach my residents. Sometimes when I'm attending, I feel like medically there is so much opportunity for them to learn from others that I sometimes wonder, "What am I really offering?" What I try to offer them is an approach to the patient and just what it takes to be a good doctor. I think that teaching them how to apologize was a very important lesson. It was just a really great learning experience.

I think this is a pretty nurturing place. Over the years, when I've done good things and when I've taken a step in my career, I received recognition. Those words mean a lot. If I looked into my saved e-mail file, I have things from years ago. For example, one from 2003 reads, "Your chapter is superb. It's exactly what the book needs. Thank you. Thank you. Thank you." That's the kind of thing I save and save forever. I just keep that in my e-mail save file, so if I ever get depressed I can bring it up and read it.

Editor Commentary

The leaders of the medical residency program have developed a system to help the residents become successful clinicians and physician leaders. The program provides the residents with exemplary role models, resources, and processes that are aligned with the mission of partnership and collegiality. There is a long-standing tradition of nurturing, rewarding, and recognizing talents and interests. The residents are nurtured both professionally and personally. Instead of allowing them to "sink or swim," the program is purposely designed to be supportive and nurturing in a blame-free environment.

One of the obvious success factors for the medical residency program has been to make a conscious choice to select a different type of applicant. Although academic success in medical school is essential as an initial screen, the process by which they select for other important characteristics—interpersonal skills, vision, ability to work with others—has created and continues to create a unique culture.

Uncommon in many programs in the past, the approach is one where the attending physicians and more senior residents treat the new residents with kindness, compassion, and respect. As the residents learn the more technical aspects of medical care, they are also receiving an education in how to interact with their colleagues (in nursing, research, administration, and support areas) with whom they will collaborate. They learn to be successful early on by using the resources and talents of those team members.

The residents learn that it is a privilege and a responsibility to take care of patients and families. They bond with the person not just the patient. They learn from the senior residents and faculty that the personal connection with patients is encouraged and almost expected. In fact, most residents don't wait to put these ideals into practice; they get to know their patients as people, as evidenced in many stories, including several about visiting patients in their homes.

There are numerous examples of how this supportive culture is lived and practiced every day. The stories of how the residents develop their competence and confidence in a blame-free environment are telling. The ability of the most senior doctors to benefit from insights of residents who are collaborating with researchers gives meaning to the concept of meritocracy—where good ideas can come from anyone and we can learn from each other. As medicine continues to migrate to a team-based, collaborative field, the physicians from the Brigham are leading the way.

Table 13-1 Organizational Demographics

Organization	Robert Wood Johnson University Hospital Hamilton
Location	Hamilton, NJ
Setting	Suburban
Communities served	Urban, Suburban
Type of organization	Acute Care Community Hospital
Number of beds	204
Number of FTEs	1,356
Scope of service	On-campus services include cardiac catheterization, emergency angioplasty, cardiac rehabilitation, cardiology, neurology, level II maternity, obstetrics and gynecology, occupational and corporate health, orthopedics, sleep medicine, bariatric surgery, outpatient diagnostic and pre-admission testing, PET/CT scanning, radiology, rehabilitation services, spinal surgery, surgical services, and a vascular laboratory. The campus includes a free-standing building that houses the Cancer Institute of New Jersey—Hamilton, which offers cancer treatment services.
	Off-site offerings include 86,000 square foot RWJ Hamilton Center for Health & Wellness, a medically-based fitness center that is also home to the hospital's community education program, which includes a conference center that seats 220 people along with four classrooms and a computer lab, as well as the hospital's outpatient rehabilitation program.
Organizational awards	Designated as a "Get With The Guidelines" Coronary Artery Disease(CAD) Hospital—August 2006 Awarded by the American Heart Association for continuous quality improvement for prevention of cardiovascular disease and stroke.
	Specialty Excellence Award—2006 Awarded by Healthgrades, Inc.—The award recognizes RWJ Hamilton's *Orthopedic Services* to be in the top 10% of all U.S. Hospitals
	Specialty Excellence Award—2006 Awarded by Healthgrades, Inc.—The award recognizes RWJ Hamilton's *Maternity Services* to be in the top 10% of all U.S. Hospitals
	2006 Distinguished Hospital for Clinical Excellence Award—February 2006 Awarded by Healthgrades, Inc.—RWJ Hamilton ranked among the top 10% of hospitals in the nation in eight specialty care areas by HealthGrades, a leading independent healthcare ratings company.
	Consumer Choice Award 2005/2006—September 2005—Awarded by the National Research Corporation (NRC).
Organizational awards (continued)	Quality New Jersey Governor's Award for Performance Excellence—The Gold Level—December 2004 Honored by Quality New Jersey in recognition of organizations demonstrating outstanding organizational practices and those that play a positive role in New Jersey's economy.
	Malcolm Baldrige National Quality Award—October 2004—The Baldrige Award is presented annually to U.S. organizations by the President of the United States.
	Employer of Choice—November 2003—Awarded by the Garden State Council for the Society of Human Resource Management.
	Corporate Award for Nursing Excellence—August 2003—Awarded by the New Jersey League For Nursing.
	100 Most Wired Hospitals Award—July 2003—Honored by Hospitals & Health.
Focus area	RWJ Hamilton Center for Health & Wellness

CHAPTER 13

Thinking Strategically

The stories in this chapter are the voices of the hospital CEO and her executive team, hospital staff, leadership from the Health & Wellness Center, nurses with the Shapedown program, their patients, and family members. Here are their stories.

ROBERT WOOD JOHNSON UNIVERSITY HAMILTON

Leadership Sets the Tone

The expectations of behavior here are modeled by our senior leadership.

The excellence standard is really up there. We were never going to be able to compete with other hospitals unless we developed that edge. Our CEO sets the standard; it falls right down from there, and you feel it. You feel that you have to pull your weight. The organization will give you as much as you want. If you want to grow more, they will give you the opportunity to do that. If you are happy where you are, they are happy to have you as long as you are still reaching for that higher standard.

If you don't have other people helping you, you are not going to be successful. Working as an individual is great, but you need good people around you. That's what Robert Wood Johnson does—they employ excellent people. The standards are very high, and that's why this facility is so successful. Leadership brings us along with them, and our standards are getting even higher.

The senior leadership team is very approachable. They are all known by their first names. They know the majority of the employees as well by their first names. Whether you are an employee, a director, or a manager, it doesn't matter. All employees feel that comfort level with the senior leadership.

All employee badges, right on up to administration, have our first name in bold letters and last name in small letters. It's really nice. You don't feel that barrier between the folks in the trenches and upper administration. It's a very warm, friendly environment where everyone's on the same page, and that type of attitude is what keeps me here.

Senior administration appears very real to the employees. They aren't tucked away in an office where you feel you can't come in and talk. They are out on the floors. They are talking to employees, and as a result, when it comes down to needing feedback from employees, whether it is positive or negative, staff feel comfortable communicating their issues to them.

Senior management understands that if we take the time in growing our people they are going to want this place to grow as an institution.

When our employee satisfaction scores weren't quite where administration had hoped, we got a letter at home from our CEO saying, "I'm responsible. Upper administration is responsible. We let you down. You let us know what your needs and wants were, and we didn't deliver. We're going to make a conscious effort to do that this year." To hear upper administration say something like that and make a conscious effort to make it better is a great example of taking ownership and accountability.

Two weeks ago I took my whole division out to lunch. We've been short staffed. Our census has been extremely high, and everybody had been running around. So I took them out for an extended lunch. I was able to communicate that this was a reward for doing a good job, and we were able to get to know each other outside the workplace.

I do understand what my employees are going through and support them. I practice management by walking around. They know I'm not sitting here being unaware of what's going on outside the office.

On Valentine's Day, we had a fire in our kitchen, and it was a massive mess. The fire was in one of the stoves. It happened in the morning, and we had to plan for lunch and dinner. Instantaneously, we had the dietary folks and housekeeping folks down there. The dietary department and the nutritionists were in my office within five minutes planning ahead for lunch. Immediately following that, we had a team here in the boardroom of probably 25 people.

I watched process improvement around this table making sandwiches, and I almost couldn't believe it. Somebody said, "Get a marker. Write turkey, tuna, or peanut butter at the bottom of the bag." People were going to help anyway, but what I saw happen was "what's the best way to do this?" The process improved around this table within minutes.

The whole board table was covered, and we were making tuna fish sandwiches and peanut butter and jelly sandwiches. We had people in a big assembly line. We had the CEO down that end of the table who was up to her elbows in tuna fish making sandwiches. At the finish line, they were putting things in the lunch bag with the names of the department, and they were going right out the door. It was pretty gratifying just standing in the room watching everybody wearing the gloves and aprons. It was fun too. I think we all had a little more appreciation for everybody that does this on a daily basis.

The same thing happened at dinnertime. A big group got together in our conference room, and we did dinners with food we brought in from outside. We had all of the slips for each patient's requirements, and it was an unbelievable team effort. Our CEO and our senior leaders were there with us doing everything from A through Z, including wheeling the carts out and serving the patient. It was an incredible, incredible day filled with a lot of laughs, a lot of work. I think it struck everybody in the organization how we can pull together. Everyone from A through Z can jump in and help when there is a problem or a challenge.

We had an executive compensation meeting last night. That committee of the board is my least favorite day of the year. I don't particularly like to talk about my money and my salary. I said to the board chair, "Don't you understand that for me it's not about money and what I'm paid here? It's about the people and the people I work with and relationship with the organization."

He said, "Oh, yeah. That's abundantly clear. We know that about you."

I think it's true. This place gets into the heart and soul of people, and I think that's a good thing.

As a leader, I think you have to make sure that you can remove the barriers to satisfaction. You have to make sure that there is clarity around the message that this is what the organization is here for. This is how it fits in with our mission and enables the managers to see good role models. When I'm out on the units and doing my job, I think the ownership sits on me, and they need to see the leaders as great role models as it relates to it.

When we received the Baldrige award, it felt like I was accepting on the behalf of all of our employees. We took pictures of all of the employees. We had to make an acceptance speech, and we were allowed 50 people to come into the room with us. We also got a couple of extra seats from the other organization. We couldn't get everybody in, but the 50 people all carried a blue hospital H with pictures of people in their departments. I felt like I was there with 1,800 employees. I felt like I was there with everybody. Everybody knew that they were recognized at that same moment.

At our strategic positioning plan meeting, this year we had a picture on the stage of the Baldrige Award with the 50 people with the blue Hs. I talked about how I represented those 1,800 employees and that I was really honored to work with all of them. It was a recognition that was really for the organization. It felt great! It was a truly proud moment.

Strategic Thinking

As the CEO, I play things, scenarios, in my mind. I spend more time thinking visionary and thinking about positioning.

We were thinking ourselves into a box. We were thinking that we needed to be a 100-bed hospital, and so, we needed to pare our expenses down to the absolute bone in order to be competitive. That was a very different philosophy for me. It just didn't feel right. I had seen other successful examples of organizations that had double-digit growth. They hadn't achieved that growth by cutting expenses. I said, "We need space to grow into."

The response was, "What do you mean? We don't have enough census. We don't have enough nursing support. Why would you do that when it will add to our cost?

I felt if we didn't do it we would miss our opportunity to grow. If we had success in all of the other areas, we wouldn't have the space for the patients. If our goals came to fruition, we wouldn't have places to put the patients and please the docs. It would impinge on our effectiveness in the other areas.

We felt that it may call for some real breakthrough strategies. Why not bring in an expert? Why not bring in someone from the outside to help facilitate discussions, interview people in the community, community leaders, board leadership, and our senior leadership. It was an incredible three-month process. We came up with strategic imperatives, and we moved from a position of lagging the market to leading in market share and image within the community.

Our strategic planning process is relatively robust. We involve a fair number of people: people within the organization, people from the community, people from the board, and certainly a lot of our docs. It provides a vehicle for not only communication and knowledge sharing and also ownership and engagement at the employee level.

As part of our strategic positioning plan process, we prioritize the goals and come up with five or six goals. Usually during the discussion process we've got a champion for that particular goal, someone who feels a passion around quality, service, finance, or whatever the goal is. There are 12 of us on the senior team going through this process. At the end of that process, we have this grid laid out, and we have stickies on it indicating who wants to be involved. Invariably we have too many people and too many goals, which to me means that people want more accountability and want to be a part. We never end up with a goal where somebody's out there on their own. It's a team effort.

I think that you need a leader when it comes to prioritizing. We decided to back our planning process up on the calendar. We did that in response to a very informal question: "How can we do this better next time?" Our department director pointed out, "You know. The budget goes to bed at the same time that my goals for the next year, and the organizational goals go to bed. Everything happens in that fourth quarter of the year. I'm less effective setting my budget when I haven't had a lot of time to reflect on what my individual goals are and what the organizational goals are." So we backed our planning process up. We have 25 to 30 goals on boards all across the room, and we talk about the importance of all of them. Then we begin narrowing that list down. Now we are able to give managers the goals and the priorities before they are thinking about their budget.

My department will discuss what three goals we want to commit to. We are given an opportunity to see where we can make the most difference in our specific department. I think that's rare in healthcare.

We have an Institute of Excellence, which is an all-day off-site program that we hold several times a year for the top 100 people in the organization and a few docs. Our senior team puts the day together. In the past, we've had out-side people come in, but we felt we couldn't connect; we couldn't create a safe space for people to speak up and be part of the plan. Now we limit it to peo-ple from our organization. We hear input from the various constituencies. It includes all of the senior leaders, the directors, the managers, and also staff members who are either in a supervisory role or are being developed for that role in the future. We actually decide on what direction the hospital needs to go in. It's an amazing process. All are actually involved in creating the strate-gic plan.

At our July institute, we talked about our position within this community, what we need to do to meet our objectives, and what was happening at the other organizations. There was this huge group of people in attendance, and I don't think there was one individual that didn't speak. We made sure that we got input from absolutely everybody; our organization is good at that. We reinvented the key sections of our strategic positioning plan. We talked about each of our competitors and listed what their strengths were, and we had a meaningful dialogue. We talked about what our roles should be, and we ended up the day with a strategic positioning plan in place. We just felt the spirit of the day. Afterward, hearing it being replayed by individuals who had come to healthcare from other industries—it was a great moment.

We've been struggling with an overwhelming volume in our emergency department, and as a result, we're holding patients while they wait for beds. It's a real stressor for the whole organization. Last year, we didn't make a lot of headway in solving that problem.

We're growing as an organization much faster than our competitors, and we are gaining market share. It's wonderful that patients from the area want to come here, but we needed to solve this problem because we're really dissatisfy-ing patients and employees when we don't have enough space for patients to move to. I wouldn't want a hallway bed, nor would I want to wait in the emer-gency room for a stretcher for a period of time.

We have had various teams working on things, and although they've had successes, we just couldn't stay ahead of it. A couple of weeks ago I asked the senior team to work very hard together to take a fresh look at the situation: "What are some action steps that we can just do to make this better?" We need to assist those teams and break down barriers that they may not see. We've got to put a whole sense of energy to it.

Several groups met, and we created an action sheet and a sense of consen-sus and ownership. There was a burst of progress right after that. We saw a dif-ferent kind of team coming together. Maybe there is a lesson there: When teams work on things for an extended period of time, it's hard to see incremental progress. It is better to shift the energy by changing team members, and then there is a boost.

I'm a nurse by background, and they don't teach you anything on strategic planning in nursing school. So, it was a great learning opportunity for most of us in the room to be involved at that level.

Doing it Better

Our motto is to achieve a higher standard. It's not just a high standard or an average standard. We have the opportunity to work at the highest standard.

The expectation is that we are empowered. If you are looking to improve something, you automatically have support to do that.

We've learned so many lessons about listening to each other and working together as a team so that we can all be better. Collectively, we're better because we listen to each other. We continue to ask that question, "How do we do this better?" It sounds like such a little question, but it's so powerful. It's given us the ability to look at processes and many other things. It's fueled our passion.

It's the commitment to quality, the passion for serving people and the processes by which we run the organization. When you combine those elements, you can break through anything.

This is one of the most challenging hospitals to work at. If you are not a hard worker and if you are not striving for excellence, you are not going to last here at Hamilton. I think the word "excellence" says it all. You can see that we change a lot here. You have to be willing to change and adapt to all the changes to work here.

You know we are held to a higher standard. You can't give yourself this simple little goal. It has to be a higher level goal. That gives you something to really work toward and to feel accountable for and to feel proud about at the end of the year when you've achieved it. You know we really impacted something; if we hadn't done this, people would not have reached their goal.

I had an individual who always liked to think out of the box. She and I talked often about, "All right. Who should we bring in? Who should we add to that group to fuel it?" We added some people to the patient satisfaction group that never were involved with patient satisfaction—food service, environmental services—those departments that aren't necessarily front line on patient satisfaction. They caught the bug, caught the fire so to speak.

As a group of senior leaders and management, we tried to develop work standards, and we bombed. It didn't work. Since we are always saying, "How can we do things better?" we took it to the employees. We asked them, "What are the standards that you feel people at RWJ need to live by?" So the employees that work here every day created these standards. They looked at everyday work habits to arrive at what are the expectations of people who work here. They helped roll out the standards to their front-line staff that they work with every day.

Managing Up

We like to send personal notes to people at their homes. A while back we decided that every director and everybody in senior leadership needed to fit that into their schedule. We had great intentions, but it just got shelved to the last thing we did. So we set up a process where, a third of the directors every week would get an e-mail from my executive assistant, which asked them to recognize somebody within the organization. The recognition process is called managing-up. They were to tell the story of something they saw that was fantastic. After receiving the e-mail, we then write the personal letters. The employees love it. The directors love it. I do the same with the board of trustees. It's a real positive thing. At the end of every quarter, every department gets a listing of managing-up letters so that it's tied right into the evaluation.

I wrote an employee a letter about how he really helped out a process. It happened to come to him right before Thanksgiving. He shared it at the Thanksgiving meal with his entire extended family and posted it in his dining room. He came in to work absolutely beaming. You underestimate the impact it can have not only on him, but also his whole family. You just have this vision of him boasting about how he was recognized. It makes you feel good that you conveyed to him, his wife, and his kids that he does a great job. You don't usually share your performance evaluations with your family over Thanksgiving dinner.

We have to give an example of what an employee did. A handwritten note card then goes out from the senior leadership team to that employee saying, "Thank you so much for doing X, Y, and Z. We appreciate it." The employees are thrilled with them. They bring the notes in saying, "Look what the CEO sent me. Look what the CFO sent in."

It makes you feel good as a person just to have somebody say thank you. I got a form thank you letter from the organization, and then when I read down there was a handwritten note at the bottom from our CEO. It said, "Thank you. It is very nice of you to contribute to the hospital." I'm not sure every letter in the hospital got a little note from the CEO, but that just made me feel great as a person knowing that I was recognized all of the way to the top.

Recently, we had a snowstorm. I live close, so I was here. We needed to pick up some key employees. When I turned around, my second in command was here. He assembled a caravan of four-wheel drive vehicles, assembled the staff. We had MapQuest running at the security command post identifying various routes and trying to batch the locations of employees' homes so that we could get them in here. It went off without a hitch. He really kicked it up a notch so I managed him up. When he received the "wow" letter he came in and said, "Thank you, but on the other hand you really didn't have to do this."

I got our outpatient center in the hospital accredited in the three different categories: general nuclear, nuclear cardiology, and PET. We are the only hospital in the state with that distinction. I got a thank you from my director. Things had quieted down, and I almost forgot about it. Then I got a handwritten letter at home from our CEO thanking me for what I had done. It was really warming to know that the top dog in the institution knew that the little dog had a hand in getting this achievement.

Not only is administration aware of what you did, but also they take the time to recognize it, and I know I am not the only employee doing good things in the institution; however, they took the time to recognize me and they take the time to do this for others. I imagine they spend a good part of their day writing these notes from the heart. They genuinely appreciate employees and I find that very, very rewarding.

My husband received a thank you note at our home from our CEO. It was at a time when we were at the hospital long hours working on a project. The note said, "Thanks. I know what it must be like to have your spouse away from home so many hours." I thought that was great. Personally, that's one thing I'll never forget.

Believing in People

I was just named "Employee of the Quarter," and that gives me a good incentive to work harder. All of these little things really make you feel good and make you want to keep coming back. That's what I have in my department.

It is not bringing out the best in someone; it is bringing out the best of a whole bunch of people. When a pivotal figure in this organization (our COO) resigned, it was difficult for the organization. The approach that I took was to talk to everybody on the senior leadership team about throwing up the organizational chart to the wind. "If you were redesigning that Org Chart, what would you want? What do you want a piece of? What do you want a piece of for your own professional development? What kind of thing thrills you? What area haven't you done?" I literally whacked up the Org Chart.

I thought the restructure was going to take a whole lot longer and that there would be things that would fall through the cracks. Instead, people who gave up areas of responsibilities to take on new areas just kind of held the hand of the person who was taking on the new responsibilities and grew.

For example, one person lost a fair number of professional services. He told me, "You know, I need some additional responsibilities down the road, and I think this area could report to me." We actually had a candid conversation about whom he should talk to about it. He had had a mentor within the organization; we do that—mentoring and pairing—and he had a good working relationship with the individual that was going to be handling some of those areas. He took on the building, clinical engineering, which was an absolute mess, environmental services, and maintenance. We have made more progress in the four months since he has had it than we had in four years before. It's like he's been rejuvenated. It's like he's jumped in the fountain of youth, and he's sprinkling it on all of us. It is beautiful.

So, I gave the COO responsibilities to 13 different people, and most people got what they wanted. The energy that I've seen since has been absolutely phenomenal. It is so beautiful. I can't tell you what it's done. It's like losing 20 pounds and feeling a new lease on life. Just feeling like you can do things that you couldn't do before.

A patient wrote in on a patient satisfaction survey, "My doc did a fantastic job." I wrote a note to the doc and shared the comment exactly, not the patient's name, but the comment exactly. I thanked him for working for our organization. One day the head of our department of surgery stopped me and said, "Can I talk to you just one minute? I can't tell you what it meant to me to get your letter about the patient. I felt like I'm not just sitting around, but I'm really making a positive impact on this organization." I wasn't expecting that a doc at his level would talk so from the heart about how it moved him to get that communication. It was a different validity, not just the validity we get from the patient saying it. I intensified the communication.

At another facility I was at, the CEO didn't know who we were as we passed in the hallway and God forbid I ever called him by his first name. Here, within the first week, our CEO came to see me, and she called me by my name and introduced herself by her first name. She knew who I was even though I'm low on the chain and I'm newly employed.

I think it's important that Robert Wood values their employees very much. They offer an employee wellness program. They help employees reduce their stress by offering chair massages and other good programs, and they value their employees. I have worked in many different places, and I have to say that this is the best place I've ever worked.

Every one of these nurse educators gets an opportunity to be in the public eye. We put them in our advertising, in our daily newspaper, and in our quarterly newsletter. People in the community know not only their names, but recognize their faces. Our patients are comfortable coming here because they know the nurses. They know the community education staff, and they feel at home.

One day a community member arrived at community education in a wheelchair. I carried her books and went out of my way to make sure that she got in the door and was comfortable. I just thought I was doing my job. Because of that, this person came back for two or three other community education lectures. A week later she wrote our CEO a letter saying that this was the first time that she'd been out of her home in 13 years. She had always felt uncomfortable and unable to come to any of our events. In the letter, she mentioned how I made her feel so special and took care of her. A week later I had a note in the mail from the CEO thanking me for that.

We have an employee satisfaction committee that was formed because our employee satisfaction survey at the time was not too good. Senior management wanted a group of cross-departmental employees to come together behind closed doors with the CEO to talk about the issues. Housekeeping, security, maternity nursing, days, nights, weekends—we are all represented. We make decisions right there if we can. The CEO sits right at the front of the table, and she is able to sometimes make immediate decisions like all right it's going to happen now. About the bigger decisions, she'll say, "It's going to have to go to the board."

A big thing we talked about was benefits; however, we were able to make the decision that would best meet the needs of most of the employees here, and we were real proud of it. In fact, because of this committee, we won an award, New Jersey Business and Industry Employee of the Year. The entire committee was invited to go to the award ceremony in Princeton. They bought our tickets and really gave us all of the accountability for a lot of the work that we did. Not everybody would have taken that kind of initiative to give the glory to other people.

At the quarterly employee forum run by senior leadership, the directors are asked to "wow" an employee during the meetings. So, quarterly, 25 different individuals get "wowed" for something that they've done. A director will get up and say, "I'm wowing so and so for her fantastic collections in Medicare" or whatever the case may be. So, the employee is recognized in front of probably 75 other employees.

At our employee forums, meetings that the CEO has quarterly for the staff, we get an opportunity to "wow" one of our staff members or a co-worker. Following that example, at my staff meetings every month, I "wow" one of the employees on that level for something they've done that month in the department.

At the quarterly staff meetings, the CEO goes over our values and our missions. There is a "wow" portion where different directors recognize employees who have done something exceptional. These employees are invited to the meeting, and they are given a little token of appreciation either a free lunch or a gift certificate. Personally, I've been recognized a couple of times. It makes you feel that you contributed above and beyond, and it just feels good for them to say thank you.

As an employee, my director a few times has recognized me, which is nice. I consider it just doing my job, but it's nice to know that he appreciates it. I'll get movie tickets or basketball tickets, and now and then we have that "customer service cash" that you can save up and get different things with.

When I usually do "wows," I try to do them outside of my division because I think it's important too that you don't always pick your own people, but I just didn't think that there was anybody else more worthy of that acknowledgment at that time. I thought it was well deserved.

I do a lot of work for strategic planning maps, and one day our CEO picked up the phone and said, "I want to invite you to the strategic planning board meeting in 10 minutes. Do you want to come?" I was scared out of my mind. They publicly acknowledged all of the work that I did, and I mean that was awesome.

I travel over an hour to get here and coming down the highway they have a Malcolm Baldrige billboard on this huge pole that announces we got the award. I sent a little e-mail to my boss saying this was really gratifying to see that and I'm kind of proud to work here. My boss forwarded that e-mail to our CEO, and I got an e-mail from her saying, "Oh, that's great. I missed it. Where is it? I'm so glad that it made you feel that way." It's really good.

I was actually invited to go to Washington to speak at the Quest conference and the award ceremony. I was just a staff member attending with directors and senior leadership. You know when you are sitting in that room with Dick Cheney up there it was so exciting. That's how they feel; they really want to thank you. They really want to give you that extra, and it makes you want to do it again.

I've noticed in a lot of employees a lack of self-esteem. One employee said, "We are only housekeepers." I said, "No, you're not only a housekeeper. You are as key as everybody else in making the hospital work. Now tell me what are the issues to make you more efficient?" I found out that if there's a clogged sink or a clogged toilet they have to call Maintenance. It means they can't clean the sink, and they can't clean the toilet. It delays them with that bathroom. I said, "Why do you have to call maintenance?"

"Because that's the way it's always been."

I said, "What would help you?"

They said, "We would like plungers."

"That's it?"

"Yes, we want plungers."

I called their director and said, "I absolutely can't believe this. I'll go to the dollar store if you don't. Order a case of plungers and put one on every cart."

What I want to do is get the best and greatest ideas out of the people I have assembled around me. I want to make sure that I've got the right people that can fix this, and I also want to make sure that I've created the environment where they understand why we need to do it, why it's important, and get everybody on board toward a common goal.

There's always that curve of people where the front line says, "Not only can we do this, but I can make it better than what you thought it was going to be." Then you've got the middle crew saying, "Yup, I'll do it. It's probably right." Then you've got the people who say, "Not over my dead body." As a leader, you feed each of those groups differently. For the people on that leading edge who are really excited, you make sure that you break down any barrier that they might have in going forward. I think the middle people you want to get them relating to those people on that front end as much as possible just to feel that spirit. Marrying those leading edge people with people in the middle created that synergy and kind of pulled the other group along.

One day my mom called me and said, "I got a call from a friend who was watching C-SPAN today, and you were on it! Your dad and I turned on the TV, and you and your hospital were on." This was during the anthrax crisis. We did not have a lot of information about what the level of exposure was or what that meant. We just knew that there were 1,400 employees at the post office around the corner who were very concerned, very upset.

There wasn't enough time to find out from CDC in Atlanta or even from the Health Department in Trenton what the proper protocol was. Most of us were here for four or five days straight, processing the workers, getting them registered, getting them seen by a doctor, getting them seen by a pharmacist, and having medications dispensed.

This organization pulled together at a time of crisis and put something together that may not have been perfect; in hindsight, there are lessons we could have learned from how we set that up, but it was pretty darn good. I was just so proud of the way the hospital was able to mobilize in such a short period of time. It happened in our community. It happened here in Hamilton, and we are the health resource for Hamilton. We felt the need and an obligation to respond to that. We didn't have anybody in New Jersey die.

We had no cases of the inhalation of anthrax. What does that say about our docs, about our employees?

Coaching and Being Coached

On the executive team, two of us have been together for eight years. The two newest people have been with us four or five years, but the core players on the senior team have been together for the entire eight years. That's a good amount of time. When you think that the average hospital CEO for a community hospital is four years, we've got double that, so we know each other well. We kind of fill in the gaps that way. We don't have to be perfect all the day. It is okay to say, "I could have done this better. I really could have done this better. Help me figure out what I need to do next time." We are not all experts in the same thing; we have to rely on each other.

One of my directors recently became an organizational superstar and really jumped ahead. It started when I asked him, "What do you see ahead of you? What would you like from me? How can I help you get there?" He wanted me to set expectations and timeframes, to maintain an open line of communication. He wanted me to give him not only the positive pat on the back, but if he was not meeting expectations, he wanted that feedback too.

We sat down, and I said, "We need to get your scores above 90% by the end of the year. How can we get there?" Together, we developed a comprehensive vision of where the department was going and set target turnaround times. Then I asked him, "What do you need to make this succeed?" He sees that I'm supporting him and that I'm dead serious about it. The team knows they have management support and I have empowered this director to make it happen.

He was a true diamond in the rough, but he didn't have the leadership to bring him forward into what he really could become. My work with him empowered him, kicked it up a notch, and he became one of our superstars.

I probably model a lot of my management skills and style after my previous boss. She allowed me the independence to go ahead and set the goals and expectations. She told me what she needed and when she needed it and that she would be there to support me, and that's what she did. I'm not an individual that needs to be micro managed. Just tell me what you need and I'll get it done. So with that, I tried the same approach in managing my directors.

With some of them, it worked; with others, it didn't. You have to be able to read the individual.

I was a narrow-minded director at the time, and I was opposed to bringing in cardiac rehab. I was saying, "Why would we want to get into this business?" It's a money loser. Why are we bringing on a service that we know will not make money? My boss had me sit down, and she told me to look at the big picture and don't just look at what was in front of me. She said, "This a service that will expand our product line. Right now we are losing some patients to other hospitals. Sure, you have to stay focused and keep this on the radar screen because we don't want it to take too much of a bath, but I want you to come up with a way to do it and cover our costs so we won't lose money."

Now I could see. I realized there was another side to this. I needed to become more open minded and look at this. It made sense. When a patient comes out of cardiac catheterization or angioplasty, they are going to need rehab services. It would also help to grow some of our outpatient services—echocardiogram, stresses, the labs—so it made sense. It also helped to recruit some other physicians in and bring patients in from other facilities. It was an "aha" moment for me.

Last year we had administrative residents. They had completed their master's degree, and two of those individuals took turns and spent three months with us. Both of those individuals wanted to come to our Institute of Excellence. I believe I saw that Institute of Excellence differently because of their observations, their input, and their sharing it with me.

When I was at other organizations, the executive team wasn't the healthiest environment to be in. There was a lot of backbiting and lot of stepping on each other, and it wasn't particularly healthy. So I thought that kind of thing must go on here, too. When the COO and I had a couple of difficult moments, I perceived it as the two of us butting heads. I think perhaps she was just trying to solve problems, and maybe I didn't respond as well as I could have.

Anyway, we had a couple of tough moments. It wasn't until one day she asked me to step into her office and said, "I don't think we are working together very well. How can we work better together?" It was a light-bulb moment for me when I realized she was sincere. She wasn't telling me "I don't think we're working well together so I'm going to tell the CEO you should go." Instead, she was saying, "How can we work better together?" It was at that moment I realized she's really trying to help me help her. We had a frank discussion about what I thought I needed from her from a communication standpoint. For the next four years I couldn't have worked better with anyone else. I think the world of her. It was a turning point for me.

I have a director who had a lot of problems in his area; cost overruns, FTEs, low patient satisfaction, and his employee satisfaction scores were the lowest in the hospital. He had an excuse for everything. Right off I asked him, "Do you want to stay here? Right now you are sending me the message that you don't want to be here. I'm not going to waste my energy with you if you don't want to be here."

I laid everything down. I let him know how others were looking at him. I think in his mind that was the "aha" moment. It was a real eye opener. We sat down, and we addressed every single item. We set objectives and put times against them. I told him which items needed to be turned around in 90 days. I needed to be specific. We had an action plan for each objective, and we met daily.

When I started getting feedback from others—his employees, other directors, other co-workers, physicians—I knew things were improving. At the end of the 90 days, we more or less tongue in cheek shook hands, introduced ourselves, and we started fresh. A few months after that 90-day period, his department took on the introduction of a new program. The implementation took a full year and was only possible because of the changes he made in his behavior and the close relationship he and I had developed.

Recently I had an opportunity to create a new position in the organization and promote one of my directors into that group. We created a new title called executive director, and we did this at a few places throughout the organization. The person who runs my patient accounting department does a good job, and she models the right behaviors for directors on an everyday basis. She is very much in tune to the goals of the organization and how we operate. She's a terrific role model for that. So we offered her the chance to move up in the organization. I offered her the chance to go on a two-year intensive at the Advisory Board for Managerial Development. Just recently I hired an executive director of finance, and I chose her to mentor the new person over the next 90 days about life at Hamilton and how we do things.

Acting Independently

It's a very short trip from making the decision that you need to improve something to being empowered to do it.

What attracted me to RWJ was the speed at which decisions can be made and the agility in changing things to better affect our bottom line and our business.

There's no artificial barrier or limitation on the way you can go about doing your job.

In collecting information on patient care, I noticed that people were documenting the time something took place based on their wrist watch, the clock on the wall, or the time stamp on a piece of equipment, and none of those was synchronized. It was impossible to accurately say how many minutes had lapsed from the time the patient entered the hospital until A, B, or C had happened. This was important to know since we were trying to improve some processes. So I brought this to the attention of a couple of people, and they said, "Okay, go ahead synchronize the clocks." I was given ownership of that. It involved multiple departments, and I didn't have any red tape to run through to get it done. You have that confidence that if you are looking to improve something you automatically have support to do it, even if you are crossing departments.

We were working toward achieving one simple thing, which was "what time is it?" It was a really cool thing to see happen. Whatever I needed to do I had decision rights to do it. I was calling people in clinical engineering who are much more senior to me saying, "Hi, we need to meet to figure out why all the computers in the hospital give different times. It was an interesting example of what seemed to be a little problem that actually was so layered, and as long as I presented a clear rational that was patient centered, nobody questioned me. I had decision rights across all departments.

The process of fixing the clocks didn't really take very long. It made me feel very efficient. I didn't have any red tape to run through. I didn't feel like I had to be perfect at it either because other people were giving me feedback. I wasn't alone and everybody helped. I didn't have to think much about it actually it was just getting done.

Every Thursday morning we have a stroke risk assessment, blood pressure, and cholesterol screening for the community. A couple of weeks ago we had an older woman who barely spoke English. I believe she was close to 90, a little Italian lady. She came in, and her blood pressure was sky high. The nurse educator sat down with this lady to find out what was going on. She was symptomatic. She had tingling down her left side; it seemed like she was really on the verge of having a major event. She finally admitted to the nurse that she couldn't afford her blood pressure medication anymore, and so, she was taking her daughter's medication. She wasn't even sure what it was. She just knew that it was medicine, and she was taking it. Well, this nurse educator spent the next two hours with this community member. She called 911, got her to the emergency room, got her family to the emergency room, and contacted the family practitioner and nurse manager at that doctor's office to work with that family to get this woman the medication that she needed.

When a participant from one of our colorectal cancer screenings had results come back positive, I notified her by phone. She said that she had a history of a polyp. She was very concerned about it. She had decided to follow-up herself with another gastroenterologist. She had an appointment with a gastroenterologist, but it wasn't until the end of the next month. When she came in to pick up her letter, she looked very upset, so I called the office manager at her doctor's office. They said that they couldn't move her up unless there was a cancellation because the physician was booked. I called the office manager, and I told her the history and that the patient really needed to have that appointment moved up. She got an appointment the next day to be checked by the physician. The patient was just so grateful, and it was so wonderful that I could do that for her.

New Employees

We had about seven or eight people step up to help improve the process of orientation. Five were selected to come with me to Atlanta and spend a couple of days at the Ritz going through their training program. The biggest thing I remember hearing was, "At Ritz Carlton, we use orientation for people to become part of our organization not simply learn about our organization." That connected with the team and me. We came back, and we completely revised our orientation program and built it around our five-star standards. We made it much more interactive. There are skits, role plays, and all kinds of things going on so that when that day is done, that group of people knows what customer service looks like for our organization. They know what treating each other as co-workers looks like in our organization and what the expectations are.

As a result of the revised orientation, we took our 90-day turnover from almost 30% down to about 12%. It saved a lot of money for the organization, led to better services to our patients and our communities, and means less hiring we have to do. It was a big deal.

After redesigning our orientation process, our new employees have an infusion of Hamilton culture under their skin. During orientation, we literally put down a red carpet for everyone coming in to walk across. We show what teamwork means. We show what commitment to the customer looks like and what courtesy and etiquette mean to us at Robert Wood. As a new employee, you know from day one what's important to us.

We hire people expecting that they will be held accountable to our five-star service standards. It is expected that when I see someone in the hallway, and I make eye contact and smile that they will do the same. If a new employee does not do that at orientation, they are told that they will. We tell them that it won't be long until they are smiling until it hurts. We are all held to the same standards.

Our CEO does the welcoming remarks for the new employee orientation. It is important for new employees to see the CEO on the first day of employment. Management participates in the entire orientation. So the new employees see that right from the very beginning we are engaged in their employment and that they are important to us.

We tell new employees during orientation, "If there's a lost patient, take them where they need to go. Don't give them directions. Walk them to their destination." We show them that, as the management team, we are committed to their taking care of the patient. Make the patient number one.

We put "hands" on their badge to show that they are a new employee. It signifies to others to lend a helping hand. One day there was a new physician walking around the hall aimlessly. A housekeeper said, "Doc, are you lost? Let me help you get where you need to go." The doc said, "I really like this place. I think I'm keeping these hands on my badge forever."

When I was lucky enough to have an interview here a little over 18 months ago, I came in the front door, and of course, it was very scary and terrifying. I went to the front desk and told them who I was, and immediately a greeter came up to me. She said that she would take me through the many hallways and corridors to where I needed to go. I was just shocked and delighted to meet her. The way that she treated me, a total stranger who may or may not continue and be a part of the organization, was surprising. I had never run into anything like that. That attitude of outreach and caring continues to be expressed to me as a still fairly new employee—all of the way from our CEO to every new person I meet.

When I came in for my first face-to-face interview, I met with members of senior management and with the director who would be reporting to me.

They were soliciting her feedback about a potential new boss. I thought that just spoke volumes about the administrations' trust and commitment to their people. At that point, I knew if I was offered the job I was going to take it.

I think many institutions say that they have great teamwork. Even though they say they have teamwork they really function in silos, except when there is crisis. I don't see that here. I think one of the main reasons for this is that they are very selective about who they hire into management roles. They are not hiring people solely based on their credentials.

Engaging Staff

Our employees are informed and therefore engaged.

We have communication boards, and we have meeting platforms with departments and their direct supervisors. The meetings involve the CEO and the senior leadership group, and they are meant to provide information to the staff. *Hospital Highlights* provides information about what's going on within the organization. "News to Know" gives department updates, and information is always available on our intranet. We have a variety of committee structures that we encourage staff to participate on. All of this creates a circular, very tight process. Information flows downward, and information comes back up. We get a lot of valuable feedback through all these different communication strategies and modalities. The information that flows upward through the organization is what helps us adjust, be agile, and realign or re-navigate our course to make sure that we are moving in the right direction.

"News to Know" is a communication tool that is routinely available every day in every department in the morning and afternoon. It reports what's happening in the hospital. There might be a special event or special screening offered to employees that day. It also provides the opportunity to post departmental news. Messages are disseminated quickly rather than waiting until monthly staff meetings or quarterly forums. That's been a definite improvement.

The hospital is focused very much on service to the community and to patients. Whenever there is a problem, the response is proactive. "Okay, this is the situation. These are the problems, and these are the potential solutions." Our input into finding the solution is always invited.

It's great to be involved in an organization where you can see that you're a part of implementing change. You're a part of making growth happen.

One of my most memorable experiences in this process of developing strategic goals was the "Pumpkin Bucket" exercise. At the Institute of Excellence, a leadership forum that we hold quarterly, we were prioritizing our strategic goals. We had plastic pumpkin buckets lined up, and we selected what was going to be our priority by putting little raffle tickets in various pumpkin buckets. Not only was it very educational and fun, but also we got our job done. Of course, we had to go through several reviews after that, but I thought isn't that interesting and lighthearted to take something so important and really make it a fun and memorable experience.

I'm from patient accounting, and our goal is patient cash. It ties back to the organization goal of margin management. My employees wear our goals on the back of our badges. I keep a running total of cash collected on the wall in the department and monthly I mark where we're at on the thermometer. Employees feel that they are truly engaged, that it is up to them to make this organization a success. The strategic plan is not just a book somewhere. They have a piece in working to help the organization succeed.

On the back of our badge is a card that lists the commitments I have made to help my department attain their department goal. It's something very specific, like I will answer the call bells within X period of time, or I will turn this radiology test around within X period of time. It is a measurable goal for me that will contribute to meeting their goal.

A key component of my revenue cycle was severely broken. I knew that until I got to the core of what really happens that I wouldn't be able to affect change. So I said, "Tell me what you do every day?" That was the beginning of a process flow chart that covered the boardroom wall. Then I asked, "Is this what we do every day?" Everybody agreed. "Well, why does it take so long?" Nobody said anything.

I said, "Well, how can we find out?" So we followed a days worth of charts; even with that data back up on the wall we still didn't understand why it took 10 days, but we did understand where things were coming off line. Without being critical or judgmental, this group discussion started. People talked about what they do every day and how we could make it better. They began to visualize a different way of doing the work. Now instead of being a notable poor performer the department is one of our stars.

In preparing to present our goals to the medical executive committee, I began at the front end. I had a meeting a few days before with the physician that chairs the committee so that we could go to the board together instead of me presenting alone. I built consensus with him first. We heard input from the docs that we didn't have the strategic goal prioritization right. We had placed quality at the top and patient throughput as the second priority. The consensus of that group was patient throughput should be first because it really impacted them, impacted their daily lives, and impacted the quality of the care. They said they would get to their quality objectives if we could fix the patient throughput. It was great input. They were right. We were wrong.

I think very clearly, if my reaction had been, "Thank you for your input. I'm not changing. You guys don't know the whole thing," I would have killed myself for years to come. It would have been like putting a noose around my neck and standing on the edge of a chair. I needed to engage them. I needed to have them be more involved with this strategic planning process. I needed their real input. As a result, they stepped up to the plate and gave valuable input.

Healthy Community

We can't just think about making sick people better.

The mission is pretty simple. It's excellence through service. What we're all about is making this community a better place to live. We took a narrow approach with the organization when we developed that mission statement and that mission statement says it. We're here to serve the healthcare needs of this community, to improve the health of the community

Our mission is to preserve, promote, and restore the health of the community. It's all about wellness and our community and taking care of them. We are the community.

What would I love? I would love to make a difference in central New Jersey and improve the health so that fewer people have to come into the hospital. There will be less obesity, less diabetes, less cardiovascular disease, and there will be the systems—the structures—in place so that people are really supported.

We have a pretty extensive community education outreach, and part of what we do here that's different is really focused on prevention and wellness.

When you speak to people on the outside, you hear, "The Wellness Center is a beautiful building. It's wonderful. They have all kinds of wonderful classes. They give back to the community, and it really shows." The community is just awed by it.

Our philosophy is to provide the structure, the motivation, and the support to be successful in our programs. We provide the trainers. We provide the nurses assessments and the classes. What's most important is that we follow-up. What I get out of my job is when people come into my office after they have signed up and say, "Thank you. You have changed my life. This has probably saved and extended my life."

We are actually encouraged to create and design new programs. Community health is something that is very close to my heart. It's promoted all of the time to the community. We are constantly reaching out. We provide health and wellness education to a community that is hungry for it and appreciative of it, and we have an administration that supports it 100%. It's a wonderful thing.

I really love the dedication that this hospital administration has to the community. The resources they have put in place really do serve our community. I'm from Hamilton. I was raised and went to school in Hamilton. I feel I'm here giving back to my community. I admire the administration for giving us the opportunity and the resources to do what we do in the community. I feel that our department and our organization operate as a family, and I wouldn't want to work anywhere else.

I am a therapy nurse. I do the more holistic programs of body, mind, and spirit. In the 1970s, I made up in my mind a job where I would go around to patients in the hospital who were very anxious, and in some way, I would reassure them and put their mind at ease. We didn't even have a word for it back then. When this position came up five years ago, I thought, "Oh, my goodness. This is the position I dreamed up in the '70s."

I have yet to be asked a question by a community member or a co-worker that I couldn't answer. I think that's part of building big networks and relationships with each other and community members and community agencies. We know so many other people working with the community and the services that are out there that we are able to refer people to another service to get an answer. I think we are very strong in that area.

We have several big health fairs every month. Every time we meet one new agency or one new person to add to our network, we follow-up with those people. We keep in touch and utilize them for future events. We have had people ask us how they can be a part of our future health fairs and programs—knocking on our door saying, "I want to be a part. How can I get involved with your programs? This is what I have to offer. Does it sound like something of interest?" We get those types of calls daily.

Thousands of people come to our events. We use the whole center and just spill out all over. We've been known to rent huge tents and set them up on the hospital campus. Community members come through and visit the tables and pick up information.

I have been a nurse for almost 10 years. I've worked for other big hospitals, but never have I seen the kind of rapport that a hospital has with its community as I have found here.

I've had the opportunity to see all of these changes and see the difference we've made in the community over the years. I stay at RWJ because of the changes and just how much we take care of the community and how much the community respects us also.

One of the things that I had identified as a need was training for school nurses to identify kids at risk for diabetes. I put together a group of our community educators and our diabetes educators, and we started to talk about the incidence and prevalence of diabetes in our community. At the same time, we were partnering with Bristol-Myers Squibb, doing some research on a new drug for diabetes. Someone on the team said, "Why don't we see if we can get a grant to send certified diabetic educators out to schools to teach school nurses how to identify kids at risk for diabetes."

Initially we wanted to reach everyone in Hamilton Township. Then we expanded it to everyone in the county. Forty-seven schools! The challenge was to tell such a compelling story that Bristol-Myers Squibb would give us the money that we needed to implement this program. In the ensuing months, we did just that. We wrote the grant, got the funding, and started going out to the schools.

What the team found in the first 25 schools they visited was the kids identified as at risk for diabetes were also obese. Then we needed to create an adolescent weight management program. We started with an ongoing research relationship and took that community need and energized a team. We created the internal and external resources that we needed and actually got additional funding from Bristol-Myer Squibb for a childhood obesity program.

There is a statewide initiative called the Mayors Wellness Challenge. They are now using our childhood obesity program as a model for programs they are developing for kids. New Jersey Network wants to create a statewide program on their cable station. The vision is that there will be entertaining shows about healthy eating and exercise for kids on New Jersey TV. This has the potential—this little idea that started in community education and marketing and public relations to be a national effort to fight childhood obesity and improve lives.

The school nurses do initial screenings in the schools. We also get referrals by word of mouth. We go to health fairs. We advertise. We go to doctor's offices and meet physicians. We also work with teachers. We bring teachers in to our Health and Wellness Center where our healthy cooking kitchen is just like the *Emeril Live* kitchen.

I like to tell people that we are "thinking outside the cake box." Instead of focusing on cookies, cakes, and cupcakes for holiday or birthday celebrations in the schools, we are educating teachers and school nurses to promote what we call Healthy Sunny Celebrations. These focus on activities instead of food, and when snacks are provided, they are healthy—not sugary. For me, it is so gratifying, seeing that those nurses and those teachers actually make a difference in kids' lives.

Each morning my alarm clock goes off, and even though I may still be tired, I look forward to coming to work to speak to families and children about type II diabetes, healthy food choices, and exercise.

I feel that as a small team with a demanding amount of work, we all walk the talk! The entire team is focused on the children and their families. It is a great feeling to be able to count on your co-workers to get the job done and also volunteer to work extra hours if needed. We all pull together to develop the best and most informative lesson plans that we can in order to prevent type II diabetes in children. The team is extremely knowledgeable and dependable, and I feel very lucky to be part of this team.

Shapedown

"Shapedown" is a trademark program developed by the University of California in the late '70s. It is a 10-week program for kids between the ages of 8 and 13. At RWJ, it is a free program because of a Bristol-Myers grant.

Normally, the cost for 10 weeks would be $350. Insurance doesn't cover it. We've trained to date 1,400 children, and I would say at least 400 of those are overweight. That's over one third who are overweight, and grossly overweight.

We meet once a week for about two hours. The head trainer at our Health and Wellness Center helped us develop an exercise routine for the children. The parents are encouraged to join in too. They really enjoy that, and then we go into the actual Shapedown lesson. Each week we have a different topic. One week it is portion control. Another week it is label reading and nutritional analysis.

Once every ten weeks we cook in class. We give them recipes every week to take home and try, and we don't just focus on losing weight. We do a piece on communication and self-esteem.

I tell the parents when they first call to inquire about the program, "It's not a diet." It's all about moderation. We give the kids and their parents the tools to make better healthy eating choices. It is a lifestyle change for the whole family. Parents and other siblings are required to come as well. There are so many family dynamics involved.

Participating children and their families come in for an initial interview to meet us and get familiar with the facility. I remember one boy in particular who left an impression on me. During the interview with his mother, the boy turned to his mom and told her that her palm pilot, cell phone, and computer were more important to her than he was. Mom admitted to this saying that she had a stressful job and often works when she is at home instead of cooking healthy meals and spending time with her son.

Part of the program involves the children and their parents setting goals and discussing any challenges they anticipate. The son set exercise goals and was meeting those goals weekly. He was doing a fantastic job using the treadmill his mom and dad bought.

During the fifth week of the program, I was reviewing this family's goal and challenge sheets, and I was overcome with emotion. Mom had decided to clean out the office that she had in her home and turn it into an exercise room in order to spend more time with her family. She also promised to cook healthy meals. At that moment, I knew that we had gotten through to this family and were making a positive difference in their lives.

One family signed up for the program. The first couple of weeks Dad and the older sister went through the motions because they had to be there. In about the fifth week, during an exercise on effective ways to communicate, the daughter raised her hand quickly and turned to her father and said, "Dad, I feel upset when you spend more time with my sister. Would you please spend more time with me?" From that night on, the whole family came in with smiles. The patient has lost 20 pounds and has been on TV and in the newspaper. It is really great. Since then, this family has referred two additional families to us.

Patients First

Our mission of excellence and to service is mainly focused toward the patient. In my maintenance department, patients come first. If we get a call, it could be that the patient is hot or cold. The TV's not working. The toilet needs plunging. It's always patient first. We really try to reach that excellence of service for the patient.

In the maintenance department, one of our favorite sayings is "would you do that in your house?" If it's not good enough for you, it's not good enough for the hospital. That's owning the responsibility and owning the workmanship of your job. It is part of our goal for patient satisfaction and service.

Patient satisfaction is very key here at the hospital. It's a very friendly place to work. Everybody says hello in the hallway down to the doctors, the nurses, everybody, and when you walk down the hall, if any patient or family member looks a little bit lost, an employee will stop and say, "Can I help you?" If there's a call light on somebody will stop and ask the patient, "What can I do for you?" That's patient satisfaction.

Patient satisfaction and quality are definitely number one around here, and it shows with our patients. A lot of seniors that have moved into senior complexes down by the Jersey Shore still come back here because of the care we provide. Patients travel far and wide to come here no matter where they live.

Every department is affected by the throughput initiative. During the census crisis, we were on high alert. I am part of the education group, and we moved beds. When patients needed to come out of the ER, our education department went up to the ER, and we moved them to the floor they were going to. Everybody had a role: finance, marketing, everybody, regardless of their position.

We were wearing shirts and ties, and the patient we wheeled into the room said, "You guys are the best dressed patient escorts I've ever seen." We told them we were actually directors of the department. She said, "Then why the heck are you moving patients?" We told the patient that the department was busy so we all pulled together to do whatever it took to get the patients in and comfortable. The patient replied, "That's why I love this place, and that's why I've always come to this place and no where else." That was cool.

My initial motivation in applying to become a nurse was to impact individuals in a positive way. I think that the patient satisfaction orientation at a hospital is always about the person in the bed. We're all here really to take care of the patient. So there is that constant reminder that all issues are patient satisfaction issues, from food service to every small thing. All employees feel that patient satisfaction is their personal and organizational goal.

As a nurse, you want to work at a place you feel proud of. You want to come to work and know that we're doing good work here. You want to feel that your family member could come to RWJ and that you would be comfortable with the care they received.

I remember a time when our scores weren't something you wanted to talk about. We worked so hard to get them up, and we won the Baldrige National Quality Award. We were so proud of this organization. You could feel it.

In one of the oncology units, a patient with end-stage cancer longed to visit the beach one more time. We knew that was not in the realm of possibilities, so the staff brought the beach to her. They had sand brought in. They brought in beach chairs and beach umbrellas. They made nonalcoholic beach drinks, and when they brought the patient into the room, there was beach music playing. It was one of her last memories. There was no red tape. They didn't have to go to administration for permission because they knew that if it was for the good of a patient, it was okay. That's the way we see our leadership here, as modeling the way we are supposed to be.

Editor Commentary

The commitment to a "higher standard" at Robert Wood Johnson University Hospital in Hamilton, NJ is a driving force behind the success of the organization, which culminated in 2005 with the receipt of the Malcolm Baldrige Award. Essential to this inquiry is acknowledging the successes that already exist and valuing the team's current efforts that have already produced good results, and yet, in so honoring the existing achievements, it also inspires and challenges the team to continue to move forward and get even better. Continually asking, "How can we make this better?" produces operational, financial, clinical, and service results that have been recognized as a national standard.

Despite their successes, the leadership team has courage to try new things: Splitting up the COO position, letting med execs change the goal priorities, new ED improvement team, sending a letter to employee's home about low employee satisfaction scores are a few examples. They have a willingness to be uncomfortable and to confront situations where things aren't working and make them better.

An extraordinary, visionary CEO has engaged the hearts and minds of the entire leadership team, physicians, and staff members. The language of a "higher standard" has permeated the organization, and employees at all levels use this vocabulary to speak with pride of their achievements and to motivate themselves to continue to tweak (and sometimes overhaul) their personal performance and processes throughout the organization.

Leaders throughout the organization express unwavering confidence in the ability of their staff members to continue to make improvements; they are not resting on their laurels of being told they are "already the best." Their strategy of aligning each staff member's goals with the organizational ones and having them wear them everyday on their name badge keeps the improvement agenda at the forefront of all communications. It also establishes a high level of accountability for results and expectations of goal achievement; at the same time, it creates the empowerment needed for leaders and staff to be creative and try new ideas.

A strong recognition of the importance of ongoing communication and information sharing appears vital to their success. They've developed and implemented numerous and varied communication mechanisms, including white boards, meetings, and perhaps most uniquely, twice-daily newsletters.

Leaders are role models—approachable, humble, exemplars—and yet take responsibility for the ultimate results. At the same time, they exercise great humility and make great efforts to share the recognition and awards with team members. Thank you notes are used extensively, and they work. Employees throughout RWJUH-H feel appreciated and recognized, which in turn encourages them to reach again for a new "higher standard."

CHAPTER 14

Thematic Summary

The qualitative and quantitative research conducted by the editors and the contributors reveals four prevalent themes that relate to the Healthcare Causal Flow Leadership Model: high patient satisfaction, favorable healthcare climate, supporting artifacts, and successful leadership behaviors.

HIGH PATIENT SATISFACTION

In addition to the high patient satisfaction scores reported by the masterpiece organizations, we heard much anecdotal evidence of satisfied patients during the interviews. Even when they were frightened, facing a poor prognosis, or surrounded by a busy healthcare environment, patients made positive comments. They stated that they were "truly cared about," were "at a hotel," encountered "no surprises, and the "staff was wonderful." It is apparent through the stories from these satisfied patients that they were part of a healthcare climate that fostered positive staff/patient encounters. For example,

Patient Comments

"It's just the way they handle you, the way they move around, and the caring conversations they have with you."

"She talked with me everyday and truly cared about me. She was so nice to my grandson and really improved my health by creating a happy environment."

"I really appreciated the housekeeper I had on Sunday. She went and bought me a paper. That was so nice of her. I felt as if I were in a hotel."

"The nurse was very good. She is very calm and does a great job of answering my questions."

"Everyone, from the volunteers at the front of the hospital to the physicians and nurses, have smiles on their faces, and a very, very positive attitude."

"Doc, you are not going to believe this. I got my fingernails back. I'm going to come up later this week and show you."

FAVORABLE HEALTHCARE CLIMATE

The climate includes much more than employee satisfaction (Figure 3-3). Employees worked together as a team, had clear direction, and were recognized and rewarded for their efforts. They also felt a sense of pride in their work and ultimately produced a culture of greater accountability and dedication to patients. They were motivated to do the right thing and to continuously do better.

The above-average Healthcare Climate Survey scores (Figure 3-4) and the staff stories from the masterpiece organizations contain numerous examples from employees who feel energized about the environment they work in. For example,

Employee Comments

"I admire my manager. He speaks clearly about the values that have driven our success. When he wants us to work hard, we see him working hard. When he tells us to be responsive, we see him clearly setting the standard. He believes in us and we believe in him."

"We're not just good to our patients; we treat one another with loving care also. We nicknamed one of our nurse directors the *Queen of Notes*. She sends notes of recognition, thanks, encouragement, praise, and congratulations. You name it and she sends it—to everyone, not just employees."

"I was given ownership of that. It involved multiple departments, and I didn't have any red tape to run through to get it done. You have that confidence that if you are looking to improve something you automatically have support to do it, even if you are crossing departments."

"I feel that everybody rolls up their sleeves and pitches in when the going gets tough. Often times they step out of their job to help."

"My organization asks a lot of me. I would do anything for them, though."

"I love what I am doing. This community is important to me. We are creating a healthcare system for the next generation."

SUPPORTING ARTIFACTS

The high patient satisfaction and the favorable climate were not achieved solely by successful leadership competencies and style. We saw another variable in the causal flow that was vital in enabling the masterpiece leader. We refer to this variable as an *artifact.*

Definition

In the Healthcare Causal Flow Leadership Model (Figure 14-1), we use the term artifacts to represent *the unique processes or support structures that enable employee behaviors.* Although they are tangible and concrete and are often accompanied by specific tools, artifacts are not inanimate. They are constantly in motion within the organization.

We saw many examples of artifacts that the masterpiece organizations have built into their everyday work structure. A few examples of the artifact tools are thank you notes to patients, follow-up telephone calls, managing-up recognition, a 2:55 checkout greeting, mission moments, and service hero stories. However, these are not the artifacts per se. It is the 10-step process (Figure 14-2) of which the tools are a part of, that makes them true artifact.

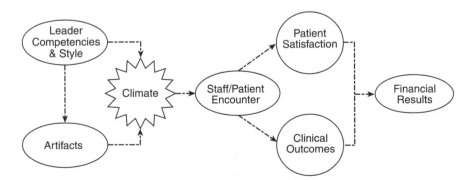

FIGURE 14-1   Healthcare Causal Flow Leadership Model. Source: Published by the editor at UMMC. Adapted from the UMMC-Hay McBer Causal Leadership Model, 1998.

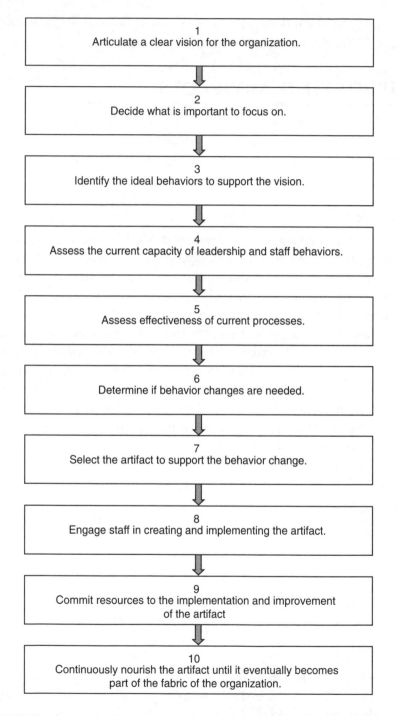

FIGURE 14-2 Ten-Step Process for Leaders to Identify and Implement Artifacts

Function

We observed artifacts that worked well at all levels of the organization. They allowed staff to do their jobs well and as a result, the staff functioned better as a team, felt recognized for their contributions, and had a sense of pride.

Artifacts were part of the daily routine that supported behavior changes. They minimized the risk of failure. Until new behaviors become part of a person's daily routine, they may not be sustained or utilized during busy or critical situations. Artifacts helped shift the thinking and supported the new behaviors until they became natural in all situations.

Artifacts also allowed leaders to try new behaviors that they might not otherwise attempt for fear of failure. It is this risk of failure that may keep some from trying new ways of leading: especially those in healthcare who work in a culture of minimizing risk.

Examples

Artifacts also helped individuals understand abstract concepts and theories by making them concrete. For example, the executive leadership team at one masterpiece organization talked about making an effort to spend more time recognizing staff. They decided everybody in senior leadership should send personal thank you notes to employees' homes. When this task "fell through the cracks," they developed a unique process, or artifact, they call "managing up." The first part of this artifact is the unique process that involves leaders sending an e-mail to their boss in which they recognize and compliment one of their staff members. The boss then sends a follow-up letter to the staff member's home. The second part is the supporting structures, namely, the weekly reminder that leaders receive from an administrative assistant to "mange someone up" and the database that contains employee home addresses. This weekly process personally rewards, publicly recognizes, and permanently documents employee actions. As reported, "The employees love it. The directors love it. It's a real positive thing."

Another organization wanted their patients to feel a personal connection with the staff as one component of their Five Star Service initiative. They created a unique process where each patient would receive a thank you card personally signed by each staff member they interacted with. This artifact forces the staff members to connect with the patients on a personal level; thus, they will have something personal to write on that note. It has become "part of the staff's being, their belief system, and their value structure. They own it." The leadership reports, "They would be hard pressed if you brought a manager in who tried to stop them from doing it." As a result, we heard patients give high praise for the caring staff. One patient said on admission, "Hi everybody. I'm looking forward to getting my little message."

SUCCESSFUL LEADERSHIP

The model that we saw emerging is one of leaders who are very comfortable with what we refer to as an interactive power and is a form of servant leadership. The masterpiece leaders see themselves as the leader–coach first and leader–expert second. They spend less time analyzing and trying to fix current problems but instead focus on leading, developing, and coaching others and focusing on positive ways to do things better. We have seen examples where masterpiece senior executives spend time in staff meetings asking managers and directors specific questions such as the following: "Who have you coached lately? How is that working? Who have you recognized? What resources have you committed to make things better?" They don't spend a majority of leadership meetings on minutes and numbers and graphs; they talk about how their leaders are relating to their staff. A classic example is the CEO who structured her board meetings to include inviting staff members to tell stories. When the board asked to hear about financial results, she replied, "Well, you can read."

What we have uncovered in our research is that a successful leader needs to focus on all four of these prevalent themes to be successful. If an organization focuses on one theme exclusively they run a high likelihood of failure. The more of the four themes you focus on, the greater the likelihood of success and sustainability. A focus distributed among leadership behavior, the work climate, the supporting artifacts, and satisfied patients will inevitably lead to better clinical outcomes and good financial results.

In summary, the masterpiece leadership has achieved a sense harmony by blending art and science. They invest in artifacts that support leaders and staff; create, energize, and motivate the healthcare climate; exhibit a high level of passion, excitement, and drive to perpetuate their success; and focus on the few competencies that set them apart. The essence of that leadership is summed up nicely by one of the masterpiece leaders in the following statement:

My job is to make everybody else successful. The exciting part of my job is in the coaching, the mentoring, getting people the resources, giving them the recognition, allowing them to be creative, and allowing them to run with ideas and to take responsibility for doing things right and doing things wrong and learning from them—to create a culture that has people excited about being here.

References

Ackoff, R. (2001). Management gurus and educators. *Reflections, 2*(3), 66-67.

Argyris, C. (1986). Skilled incompetence. *Harvard Business Review, September–October,* 74-79.

Argyris, C. (1991). Teaching smart people how to learn. *Harvard Business Review, May–June,* 99-109.

Bennis, W. (1990). *Why leaders can't lead: The unconscious conspiracy continues.* San Francisco: Jossey-Bass.

Block, P. (1993), *Stewardship: Choosing service over self-interest.* San Francisco: Berrett-Koehler.

Boyatzis, R. (1982). *The competent manager: A model for effective performance.* New York: Wiley.

Brown, J., & Isaacs, D. (2005). *The world cafe: Shaping our futures through conversations that matter.* San Francisco: Berrett-Koehler.

Brown, J., & Isaacs, D. (1996–1997). Conversations as a core business process. *Systems Thinker,* 1-6.

Bunker, B. (1990). *Appreciative Management and leadership: The power of positive thought and action in organizations.* San Francisco: Jossey-Bass, Inc.

Burnham, D. (1998). The New Source of Power. *Leader to Leader, Fall (10).*

Chreniss, C., & Goleman, D. (Eds.). (2001). *The emotionally intelligent workplace.* San Francisco: Jossey-Bass.

Collins, E., & Scott, P. (1978). Everyone who makes it has a mentor. *Harvard Business Review, July–August,* 89–101.

Collins, J., & Porras, J. (1993). *Built to last: Successful habits of visionary companies.* New York: Harper Business.

Cooper, M. (1965). *The inventions of Leonardo da Vinci.* New York: The Macmillan Company.

Cooperrider, D., & Barrett, F. (2002). An exploration of the spiritual heart of human science inquiry. *Reflections, 3*(3), 56–62.

Cooperrider, D., & Whitney, D. (2005). *Appreciative inquiry: A positive revolution in change.* San Francisco: Berrett-Koehler Publishers.

Cramer, P. (2004). *Storytelling, narrative and the thematic apperception test.* New York: Gilford Publications.

Danziger, J., & Conrad III, B. (1977). Yousuf Karsh. In *Interviews with master photographers.* New York: Author, 98–111.

Davis, S. M. (1984). *Managing corporate culture.* Cambridge, MA: Author.

Denning, S. (2001). Narrative understanding. *Reflections, 3*(2), 46–53.

Denning, S. (2000). *The springboard: How storytelling ignites action in knowledge-era organizations.* Boston: Butterworth-Heinemann.

DePree, M. (1989). *Leadership is an art.* New York: Doubleday.

DePree, M. (1992). *Leadership jazz.* New York: Doubleday Currency.

Dickman, R. (2003). The four elements of every successful story. *Reflections, Vol. 4, No. 3,* 51–56.

Donnellon, A. (1996). *Team talk: The power of language in team dynamics.* Boston: Harvard Business School Press.

Drucker, P. (1992). *Managing for the future.* Oxford, UK: Butterworth Heinemann.

Forrester, J. (1965). A new corporate design. *Sloan Mangement Review, 7*(1), 5–17.

Fredrickson, B. (2003). The value of positive emotions. *American Scientist, 91, No. 4,* 330–35.

French, J., Jr., & Raven, B. (1959). The basis of social power. In D. Cartwright (Ed.), *Studies in social power.* Ann Arbor: University of Michigan Press.

Fritz, R. (1984). *The path of least resistance.* Salem, MA: DMA, Inc.

Gergen, K., Gergen, M., & Barrett, F. (2003). *Dialogue: Life and death of the organization.* Taos, NM: The Taos Institute.

Goleman, D. (1998). What makes a leader? *Harvard Business Review, November–December,* 92–102.

Goleman, D. (2000). Leadership that gets results. *Harvard Business Review, March-April,* 78–92.

Goleman, D. (1998). *Working with emotional intelligence.* New York: Bantam.

Greenleaf, R. (1998). *The power of servant-leadership.* San Francisco: Berrett-Koehler.

Hammond, S. (1996). *The thin book of appreciative inquiry.* Bend, OR: Thin Book Publishing.

Hunter, J., Schmidt, F., & Judiesch, M. (1990). Individual differences in output variability as a function of job complexity. *Journal of Applied Psychology, 75,* 28–42.

Jaworski, J. (1996). *Synchronicity: The inner path of leadership.* San Francisco: Berrett-Koehler.

Karsh: The art of the portrait. (1989). Ottawa, Canada: National Gallery of Canada.

Karsh, Y. (1957) Karsh on photographic portraiture, *Wisdom, December,* 30–31.

Karsh, Y. (1962). *In search of greatness: Reflections of Yousuf Karsh.* Toronto, Canada: University of Toronto Press.

Karsh, Y. (1971). *Karsh: Faces of our time.* Toronto, Canada: University of Toronto Press.

Karsh, Y. (2003). *A biography in images.* Boston: MFA Publications.

Kegan, R. (1994). *In over our heads: The mental demands of modern life.* Cambridge, MA: Harvard University Press.

Kelner, S. P. (1999). Organizational climate and TQM. *Journal for the Center for Quality Management, 7*(1).

Kolb, D., & Boyatzis, R. (1970). On the dynamics of the helping relationship. *Journal of Applied Behavioral Science, 6*(3), 267–289.

Kotter, J., & Heskett, J. (1992). *Corporate culture and performance.* New York: Free Press.

Litwin, G., & Stringer, R. (1968). *Motivation and organizational climate.* Boston: Harvard University Press.

MacCurdy, E. (Ed.). (1958). *The notebooks of Leonardo da Vinci* (Vol. I and II, E. MacCurdy, Trans.). New York: Reynal & Hitchcock.

Marx, R. (1982). Relapse prevention for managerial training: A model for maintenance of behavior change. *Academy of Management Journal, 35,* 828–847.

Maslow, A. (1970). *Motivation and personality.* New York: Van Nostrand Reinhold.

Maturana, H., & Bunnell, P. (2000). The biology of business: Transformation through conservation. *Reflections, 1*(1), 82–86.

McClelland, D. (1987). *Human motivation.* Cambridge, UK: Cambridge University Press.

McClelland, D. (1975). *Power: The inner experience.* New York: Irvington Publishers.

McClelland, D., & Burnham, D. (1976). Power is the great motivator. *Harvard Business Review, March–April.*

McClelland, D., & Winter, D. (1969). *Motivating economic achievement.* New York: Free Press.

McClelland, D. (1998). Identifying competencies with behavioral–event interviews. *Psychological Science, 9*(5), 331–340.

McClelland, D. (1975). *Power: The inner experience.* New York: Irvington.

McLagan, P., & Christo, N. (1995). *The age of participation: New governance for the workplace and the world.* San Francisco: Berrett-Koehler.

Murray, H. (1943). *Thematic apperception test book.* Cambridge, MA: Harvard University Press.

Nuland, S. (2000). *Leonardo da Vinci.* New York: Penguin Group.

Pelote, V., DeWitt, F., and Deyfus, C. (1992). *Measuring management's impact upon total quality.* Annual Meeting of the American Society for Training and Development. New Orleans.

Pfeffer, J. (1998). *The human equation: Building profits by putting people first.* Boston: Harvard Business School Press.

Reti, L. (Ed.). (1974). *The unknown Leonardo.* New York: McGraw-Hill Book Company.

Romei, F. (1994). *Leonardo da Vinci: Artist, inventor and scientist of the renaissance.* New York: Peter Bedrick Books.

Route, L. Pelote, V., & Mazzawi, J. (2006). Connecting with a patient in ninety seconds. In *Addressing the National Mandate for Change.* Atlanta, GA: Society for Health Systems.

Schein, E. (2001). The role of art and the artist. *Reflections, 2*(4), 81–83.

Schein, E. (1992). *Organizational culture and leadership.* San Francisco: Jossey-Bass.

Schein, E., & Bennis, W. (1965). *Personal and organizational change through group methods: The laboratory approach.* New York: Wiley.

Schneider, B. (Ed.). (1990). *Organizational climate and culture.* San Francisco: Jossey-Bass.

Senge, P., & Wheatley, M. (2001). Changing how we work together. *Refelctions, 3*(3), 63–68.

Senge, P., Scharmer, C., Jaworshi, J., & Flowers, B. (2004). *Presence: Human purpose and the field of the future.* Cambridge, MA: SoL.

Simmons, A. (2001). *The story factor: Secrets of influence of the art of storytelling.* Cambridge, MA: Perseus.

Spencer, L., & Spencer, S. (1993). *Competency at work: Models for superior performance.* New York: Wiley.

Spencer, L., Pelote, V., & Seymour, P. (1998). A Causal Model and Research Paradigm for Physicians as Leaders of Change. *New Medicine, Vol. 2,* 57–64.

Stephenson, W. (1953). *The study of behavior: Q technique and its methodology.* Chicago: University of Chicago Press.

Stringer, Robert. (2002). *Leadership and organizational climate* (1st ed.). Upper Saddle River, NJ: Author.

Strongwater, S., Pelote, V., Gaw, V., Cyr, J., & Seymour, P. (1996). Integrating work redesign and CQI. In P. Boland (Ed.), *Redesigning Healthcare Delivery* (pp. 523–544). Berkeley, CA: Boland Healthcare, Inc.

Tichy, N. (1997). *Leadership engine.* New York: Harper Collins.

Wasserman, J. (2003). *Leonardo da Vinci.* New York: Harry N. Abrams, Inc.

Weick, K. (1995). *Sense making in organizations.* Thousand Oaks, CA: Sage Publications.

Weisbord, M. (1992). *Discovering common ground.* San Francisco: Berrett-Koehler.

Wheatley, MJ., & Kellner-Rogers, M. (1996). *A simpler way.* San Francisco: Berrett-Koehler.

Wheatley, MJ. (1994). *Leadership and the new science.* San Francisco: Berrett-Koehler.

Whitney, D., & Trosten-Bloom, A. (2003). *The power of appreciative inquiry: A practical guide to positive change.* San Francisco: Berrett-Koehler Publishers.

Zimmerman, H. (1996). *Speaking, listening, understanding.* Hudson, NY: Lindisfarne Press.

Zubin, J., Eron, L., & Schumer, F. (1965). *An experimental approach to projective techniques.* New York: John Wiley & Sons, Inc.

Editor & Contributing Editor Bios

Vince Pelote, MBA

Vince Pelote, managing partner with daVinci Consulting, is a senior organizational development professional, author, researcher, and speaker. Vince has extensive experience building competency models for the selection, development, feedback, and coaching of healthcare leaders. His background includes coaching healthcare executives and physician and nurse leaders on creating engaged, energized, and motivated work environments.

As the previous Director of the Center for Organizational Learning at a leading academic medical center in Massachusetts, Vince provided executive coaching for 26 senior executives and academic chairs. He also designed leadership development strategies and programs for 250 clinical and non-clinical leaders based upon 360-degree feedback and the results of a healthcare climate survey.

Vince was the primary researcher for a leadership training grant funded by the American Society of Training & Development (ASTD). He has also been actively involved with leadership development for the University Health System Consortium (UHC) and is a founding research member of the Society for Organizational Learning (SoL). He also served as past president for ISPI and Central Mass Chapter, ASTD and has been a senior examiner for Massachusetts Quality Award.

During the past 15 years, Vince has completed more than 2,000 Behavioral Event Interviews for the purpose of conducting action-research and building competency leadership models. He is the co-author along with Dr. Steven Strongwater of *Clinical Process Redesign: A Facilitators Guide,* which is published by Jones & Bartlett.

Lynne Route, MEd RN

Lynne Route is a founding partner with daVinci Consulting. She is passionate about translating theories, methods, and practices to help others improve outcomes. Lynne works closely with a variety of clients to help them develop and implement individualized and team based learning plans. Her work includes conducting positive explorations, facilitating leadership development workshops, and presenting at national conferences. Lynne coaches new college graduates, clinical and nursing staff, and individuals in career transition.

During her 20 years experience in various clinical settings, Lynne has facilitated projects related to leadership development, service excellence, patient safety, and performance improvement. Her master's degree in Adult Education complements her nursing background by bringing expertise in adult and experiential learning, technical writing, behavioral competencies, appreciative inquiry, and social motive into the healthcare field.

Mary P. Malone, MS, JD

President, Malone Advisory Services

Mary is a passionate advocate for transforming patient and family experiences. As a catalyst, coach, and consultant, she helps healthcare leaders to integrate the patient/family perspective into both strategy development and performance improvement initiatives. She emphasizes creating and sustaining a culture of "patient-inspired excellence." Her search for best practices includes visits to more than 950 healthcare organizations.

A popular speaker and insightful strategist, Mary conducts hundreds of workshops each year and recently co-edited a book, *Making It Right: Healthcare Service Recovery Tools, Techniques and Best Practices.*

Mary received an M.S. (Health Systems Management) from Rush University and a J.D. from Notre Dame Law School. She holds a B.S. (Biology) and a B.A. (Anthropology) from the University of Notre Dame. Prior to forming her own firm in 2005, she was a senior leader at Press Ganey Associates for nearly 15 years.

Contributor Bios

Robert E. Cannon, CMC

Bob Cannon is the founder and principal of Cannon Advantage, a consulting firm focused on enhancing performance and profitability for client organizations utilizing a strength-based approach. He also provides a fresh approach to business management and marketing issues in his "Taking Aim" newsletter that is available at www.cannonadvantage.com

Bob's career includes a track record of accomplishments for Textron, AMF, Gannett, Channellock, and Meritool. He was also a founder of ToolSource.com. He holds a Master of Business degree from Gannon University, a Bachelor of Arts degree from Grove City College, and he has undertaken additional studies at the Weatherhead School of Management. Bob has also been awarded the designation of Certified Management Consultant (CMC). At this time, less than 1% of all active professional management consultants in the United States have been recognized with the CMC.

Christine R. Dreyfus, PhD

Christine Dreyfus founded Dreyfus & Associates, Inc. in 1994. Dreyfus & Associates provides organizations with the best solutions to people-related issues. Christine collaborates with clients to establish or maintain a competitive advantage through more effective use of their people. Working in partnership with Dreyfus & Associates, clients develop internal capacity to establish or improve organizational systems such as employee selection, performance management, leadership development, and succession planning.

Christine has consulted internationally for over 10 years. She has served as the associate director of the Wharton Leadership Program at the University of Pennsylvania and taught in the Wharton School MBA program. Christine received her doctorate in Organizational Behavior from Case Western Reserve University. She has collaborated with Richard Boyatzis and Daniel Goleman in their research and writing on emotional intelligence. Her current interests include career paths of women leaders and leadership in education and healthcare.

Carol Gorelick EdD, MBA

Carol is the co-founder (1991) of SOLUTIONS for Information & Management Services, a firm dedicated to supporting clients in order to bring together the best in people, processes, and technology, thus helping teams and groups improve their performance through learning. Prior to SOLUTIONS, Carol worked at Prudential Securities, American Express, American Airlines, Lufthansa, and AT&T. She has an MBA with distinction from Pace University and a doctorate from the Executive Leadership in Human Resources Development program at The George Washington University.

Carol is an adjunct associate professor in Pace University's executive MBA program and a visiting professor at the Graduate School of Business at the University of Cape Town, South Africa. She is the lead author of *Performance through Learning: Knowledge Management in Practice,* published by Butterworth-Heinemann. Carol is a Trustee at the Society for Organizational Learning and a member of the Financial Women's Association of NY.

Lolma Olson

Ms. Olson, President of Sage Consulting™, founded her company in 1994 with a profound commitment to service and healing and an unwavering dedication to improving the quality of the human experience in healthcare. Today, Ms. Olson is known for her ability to inspire, empower, and motivate people, while focusing on bottom-line results—improving performance and satisfaction. In her work with an organization, she helps leadership, staff, and physicians see the best in their people, processes, and ideas. She creates innovative strategies and programs, such as *First Touch®: Building Connections,* that help organizations build relationships and cultures of service, safety, and healing.

Ms. Olson is co-author of the best-selling book, *Achieving Impressive Customer Service: Seven Strategies for the Health Care Manager.* She earned a master's degree in Organizational Development from the California Institute for Integral Studies in San Francisco, CA.

Cheri B. Torres, MBA, MA

Cheri is a doctoral student in Educational Psychology/Collaborative Learning at the University of Tennessee and an educational/organizational consultant with MTC Associates, LLC, emphasizing sustainable, transformational learning. She has worked with hundreds of corporations, community organizations, and schools using strength-based collaborative practices to develop full engagement, shared leadership, and continuous learning to support excellence in the face of change. She has authored or co-authored numerous articles and books, including *Dynamic Relationships: Unleashing the Power of Appreciative Inquiry in Daily Living, The Appreciative Facilitator: A Handbook for Facilitators and Teachers, From Conflict to Collaboration,* and *Inspire Cooperation: Teaching Young People to Manage Conflict.* In addition, she co-designed and patented Mobile Team Challenge, an award winning, innovative portable low ropes course. Cheri is a member of the Society for Organizational Learning (SoL), the Positive Change Core (PCC), and the Association for Experiential Education (AEE).

Carolyn Rainey Weisenberger, BS, LPN

Carolyn is an educational/organizational consultant with MTC Associates, LLC. She has worked with hundreds of corporations, community organizations, and schools to develop individual and organizational excellence. Carolyn has 29 years of experience facilitating wellness and growth for others, 23 of those years in the field of experiential learning. She co-designed and patented Mobile Team Challenge; an innovative, high performance portable low ropes course and winner of the Creativity Award from the Association for Experiential Education. Carolyn uses the integration of Appreciative Inquiry, other strength-based tools, and experiential education as a dynamic process for helping clients explore best practices, discover goals and visions, build relationships, and create strategic plans for success. She co-authored *From Conflict to Collaboration* and *Inspire Cooperation: Teaching Young People to Manage Conflict.* Carolyn is a member of Association for Experiential Education, the Positive Change Core, and the American Society of Training & Development.

Susan O. Wood, MS

Susan is a principal with Corporation for Positive Change, specializing in unleashing positive change in nursing, a highly respected—and beleaguered—profession. The nursing shortage calls for a novel approach to improve retention and satisfaction. Susan partners with health care organizations to find their "positive core" and create work environments that provide quality care for patients and meet the needs of staff.

Clients include Lovelace Health Systems, University of Kentucky Hospital, The Children's Hospital of Philadelphia, and an HRSA funded project with the University of North Carolina and six rural Pennsylvania hospitals. All are initiatives to improve quality of patient service, employee satisfaction, and retention using Appreciative Inquiry. Susan has an MS degree from American University/NTL Institute for Behavioral Sciences and a BA from the University of Minnesota. She lives in Mount Gretna, PA.

Carol Ann Zulauf, EdD

Carol Ann Zulauf is an Associate Professor at Suffolk University in Boston. Carol also has her own consulting practice, specializing in leadership, emotional intelligence, team development, coaching, and systems thinking. Her clients span high tech, federal and state governmental, health care, educational, financial, and consumer product organizations. Prior work experience includes being a senior training instructor for Motorola, Inc.

Carol has many publications to her credit, including her book by Linkage, Inc., *The Big Picture: A Systems Thinking Story for Managers,* and she is a frequent presenter at regional, national, and international conferences. Carol's international experience includes teaching and research work in Belarus, Estonia, Russia, Latvia, Germany, Belgium, Amsterdam, and Australia.

INDEX